MENTORSHIP IN COMMUNITY NURSING: CHALLENGES AND OPPORTUNITIES

JUDITH CANHAM AND JOANNE BENNETT

Blackwell
Science

© 2002 by
Blackwell Science Ltd
Editorial Offices:
Osney Mead, Oxford OX2 0EL
25 John Street, London WC1N 2BS
23 Ainslie Place, Edinburgh EH3 6AJ
350 Main Street, Malden
    MA 02148 5018, USA
54 University Street, Carlton
    Victoria 3053, Australia
10, rue Casimir Delavigne
    75006 Paris, France

Other Editorial Offices:

Blackwell Wissenschafts-Verlag GmbH
Kurfürstendamm 57
10707 Berlin, Germany

Blackwell Science KK
MG Kodenmacho Building
7–10 Kodenmacho Nihombashi
Chuo-ku, Tokyo 104, Japan

Iowa State University Press
A Blackwell Science Company
2121 S. State Avenue
Ames, Iowa 50014-8300, USA

The right of the Author to be identified as the Author of this Work has been asserted in accordance with the Copyright, Designs and Patents Act 1988.

First published 2002

Set in 10/12pt Garamond Light
by DP Photosetting, Aylesbury, Bucks
Printed and bound in Great Britain by
MPG Books Ltd, Bodmin, Cornwall

The Blackwell Science logo is a trade mark of Blackwell Science Ltd, registered at the United Kingdom Trade Marks Registry

DISTRIBUTORS

Marston Book Services Ltd
PO Box 269
Abingdon
Oxon OX14 4YN
(*Orders:* Tel: 01235 465500
         Fax: 01235 465555)

USA
Blackwell Science, Inc.
Commerce Place
350 Main Street
Malden, MA 02148 5018
(*Orders:* Tel: 800 759 6102
              781 388 8250
         Fax: 781 388 8255)

Canada
Login Brothers Book Company
324 Saulteaux Crescent
Winnipeg, Manitoba R3J 3T2
(*Orders:* Tel: 204 837-2987
         Fax: 204 837-3116)

Australia
Blackwell Science Pty Ltd
54 University Street
Carlton, Victoria 3053
(*Orders:* Tel: 03 9347 0300
         Fax: 03 9347 5001)

A catalogue record for this title is available from the British Library

ISBN 0-632-05707-6

Library of Congress
Cataloging-in-Publication Data
Canham, Judith.
    Mentorship in community nursing: challenges and opportunities/Judith Canham and JoAnne Bennett.
        p. ; cm.
    Includes bibliographical references and index.
    ISBN 0-632-05707-6
    1. Community health nursing.
    2. Mentoring.   I. Bennett, Joanne.   II. Title.
        [DNLM: 1. Community Health Nursing—United States.   2. Mentors—United States.
    WY 106 C222m 2001]
    RT98 .C36 2001
    610.73'43—dc21
                            2001037814

For further information on
Blackwell Science, visit our website:
www.blackwell-science.com

Contents

Contributors   xi
Acknowledgements   xiii
Introduction   xv

Part 1: The Policy Context   **1**

1   Setting the Scene: Concepts of Specialist Practitioner and
Specialist Practice Mentor   **3**
Judith Canham
Specialist practice   3
Programme organisation to meet specialist practitioner outcomes   4
The mentor for specialist practice in community settings   6
    Case study 1.1 Moving toward good mentorship   8
    Case study 1.2 Uncovering the mysteries of specialist practice 10
Context   10

2   From Policy to Practice   **12**
Joanne Bennett
Introduction   12
The need for change   13
The development of primary care groups   14
Implications for the preparation of specialist practitioners and
    the role of the mentor   18
Summary   20

3   Maintaining and Developing Quality and Equity within
Higher Education Programmes   **21**
Mary Dunning
Introduction   21
Key quality systems   22
Quality assurance   22
Quality audit   28
Quality enhancement   29
Conclusion   30

Part 2: Theory and Practice Context   **31**

4   **Learning Approaches in the Practice Context**   **33**
Judith Canham and Sue Moore
Introduction   33
Critical thinking   34
The mentor's role   34
Competency   35
     Case study 4.1 Indentifying specialist practice competencies   36
Adult learning: andragogy   38
     Case study 4.2 Enabling the development of leadership   40
The humanistic approach   41
     Case study 4.3 Utilising educational approaches to
       facilitate learning   43
The behavioural approach   43
The cognitive approach   44
The learning environment: organising opportunities for learning   44
     Case study 4.4 Using learning opportunities   45
Students' learning styles   47
Theory-practice integration   48
The application of educational theory   49
Summary   49

5   **Reflective Practice**   **50**
Joanne Bennett
Introduction   50
Reflection   51
What is critical incident analysis?   54
     Case study 5.1 Critical incident: dysfunctional
       multi-disciplinary team work   58
Reflection on process   59

6   **Clinical Supervision for the Specialist Practitioner Student**   **62**
Peter Wilkin
Introduction   62
Educational clinical supervision   63
Prerequisites to clinical supervision   65
Power   67
Assessment and supervision   68
Training   69
The supervisory relationship   69
     Case study 6.1 Counter-transference in clinical supervision   70
Turning lived experience into learning experience   71
A reflective model for educational supervision   71
Supervision for the mentor   73
Envoi   74

7   The English National Board Higher Award:
     A Strategy for Change   **76**
     Joanne Bennett
     Introduction   76
     What is the ENB Higher Award?   76
     The process   78
     Issues for consideration   84

8   Assessment of Specialist Community Practice   **85**
     Judith Canham
     Introduction   85
     Standards of assessment   86
     Purpose of assessment   87
     Types of assessment for specialist practice   87
          Case study 8.1 Continuous assessment: a means of
               enabling development   89
     Methods of assessment   90
          Case study 8.2 Diagnostic assessment: a starting point   92
          Case study 8.3 Observation as an assessment tool   92
          Case study 8.4 A learning contract as a learning and
               assessment tool   94
     Reliability and validity   95
     Identifying the academic level of practice assessment   95
     Practice assessment   96
     Portfolio development (*Joanne Bennett*)   98
     Comment   100
     Summary   101

Part 3: Practice: Opportunities and Challenges   **103**

9   The Evidence and Research Base for Practice
     Part 1 Evidence-based practice   **105**
     Joanne Bennett
     Introduction   105
     The development of evidence-based practice   105
     Part 2 Research-minded practice and research culture   **107**
     Dr Christopher Wibberley and Linda Dack
     Introduction   107
     The meaning of research for those in practice   108
     Fostering a research culture   109
     Conclusion   110

10 General Practice Nursing   **111**
     Sarah Mattocks
     Introduction   111
     General medical practice and the role of the practice nurse   111
     Facilitating practice learning in general practice nursing   113

Case study 10.1 Arranging appropriate mentorship and placement 114
Case study 10.2 Facilitating development for an experienced
    practitioner 115
Evaluating mentorship in general practice nursing 115
Conclusion 117

11 Community Mental Health Nursing **118**
Maureen Deacon
Introduction 118
The specialist practitioner award and community mental
    health nursing 119
    Case study 11.1 Mentorship for an experienced practitioner 120
The role of the community mental health nurse 121
    Case study 11.2 Creative mentorship 122
What helps mentors carry out the role successfully? 122
Conclusion 124

12 Community Learning Disability Nursing **125**
Peggy Cooke
Introduction 125
Viability of programmes 126
The preparation of the mentor 126
    Case study 12.1 Mentorship requirements: who and where? 127
Support for the mentor 128
The student as learner 128
    Case study 12.2 Managing potential role and relationship
    conflict 129
Student learning – environment, experience and assessment 130
Student assessment 130
Conclusion 131

13 Community Children's Nursing **132**
Carole Proud
Introduction 132
Focus group 133
    Case study 13.1 Specific placements to meet learning needs:
    example 1 135
    Case study 13.2 Specific placements to meet learning needs:
    example 2 135
Conclusion 139

14 Health Visiting **140**
Joanna Bateman
Introduction 140
Health visiting: some current issues and dilemmas for mentors 141
Managing the learning experience 143

Contents

Case study 14.1 Students' experience of very different
placement   144
Case study 14.2 Managing the first few months of
the placement   145
Assessment of practice   148
Conclusion   149

15 Occupational Health Nursing   151
Jan Rose
Introduction   151
Occupational health services   152
Factors influencing the facilitation of learning in occupational
health nursing   152
Case study 15.1 Denied access to learning   154
A more positive perspective   154
Strategies for bridging the practice-theory gap in occupational
health nursing   155
Case study 15.2 Using an experiential taxonomy   157
Summary   157

16 District Nursing   159
Anne Robinson
Introduction   159
Policy context   159
Implications for district nursing   160
Challenges for the mentor   161
Case study 16.1 The need for practitioner development:
views of a nurse executive (personal medical service)   161
The teaching and learning environment   162
Case study 16.2 A student profile   162
Conclusion   165

17 School Nursing   166
Jennie Humphries
Introduction   166
The role of the school nurse specialist practitioner   166
Mentor preparation   167
Case study 17.1 Managing mentorship and existing role
commitments   168
Mentor support   168
Case study 17.2 Being a mentor and a 'student'   169
Fostering a positive student-mentor relationship   169
Case study 17.3 Enabling student self confidence   169
Facilitating the achievement of learning outcomes   170
Case study 17.4 Am I doing it right? Using a
tripartite relationship   170

Assessment   171
Strategies for student support   171
    Case study 17.5 Facilitating appropriate student support   172
Conclusion   172

18 Being a Specialist Practitioner Student   **173**
Carole Wills
Introduction   173
The practicalities of becoming a part-time student   173
Practice placement   174
Reflecting on the student role   174
University experience   175
Home life   176
The ENB Higher Award   176
Consolidated practice?   177
Back to reality   178
Supporting other specialist practitioners   178
Conclusion   179

19 Being a Mentor   **180**
Marjorie Cavanagh
Introduction   180
The learning environment   181
    Case study 19.1 Reflection: a beneficial process for student
      and mentor   185
    Case study 19.2 Reflection: enabling student progress   186
Supporting students throughout and beyond the academic year   187
Summary   187

20 Navigating Practice: Challenges and Opportunities   **188**
Joanne Bennett
Introduction   188
Reflecting on the issues   188
What are 'wicked issues'?   189
The context   191
Towards a new approach   195
Conclusion   199

21 Concluding Comments   **201**
Judith Canham and Joanne Bennett

References   203

Index   215

Contributors

Joanna Bateman B.Nurs, RGN, RHV, NDNCert, PGCE, MSc. Senior Lecturer at the Manchester Metropolitan University, Department of Health Care Studies

Joanne Bennett RGN, NDNCert, RNT, MA, BA. Principal Lecturer at the University of Northumbria at Newcastle, Division of Primary Health Care.

Judith Canham RGN, NDNCert, PGDE, DNT, MSc. Senior Lecturer at the Manchester Metropolitan University, Department of Health Care Studies

Marjorie Cavanagh RGN, NDNCert, CPT, BSc (Hons). District Nurse with Tameside and Glossop Priority and Community Services NHS Trust.

Peggy Cooke RMNS, CNMH, RNT, MA. Principal Lecturer at the Manchester Metropolitan University, Department of Health Care Studies

Linda Dack RGN, RCM, RHV, FETCert, MSc. Service Manager for Salford and Trafford NNS Trust, Community Therapies and Audiology

Maureen Deacon RMN, SRN, BA (Hons) MPhil. Senior Lecturer at the Manchester Metropolitan University, Department of Health Care Studies

Mary Dunning RGN, SCM, RNT, MA, Ded. Professor of Nursing at the University of Northumbria at Newcastle, Division of Primary Health Care

Jennie Humphries RGN, SC, RHV, SN, Cert Ed, MA. Senior Lecturer at the University of Central Lancashire, Department of Primary and Community Nursing

Sarah Mattocks RGN, PNCert, PGDE, Med, BA. Senior Lecturer at the University of Northumbria at Newcastle, Division of Primary Health Care

Sue Moore RGN, RNT, MSc. Senior Lecturer at the Manchester Metropolitan University, Department of Health Care Studies.

Carole Proud RSCN, BN, PGCE, MSc. Senior Lecturer at the University of Northumbria at Newcastle, Division of Primary Health Care

Contributors

Anne Robinson RN, NDN, HVCert, CPT, BSc (Hons), PGDE. Senior Lecturer at the University of Northumbria at Newcastle

Jan Rose RGN, RHV, OHNC, Cert Ed, MA. Now retired but continues an interest in community health care through writing

Dr Christopher Wibberley PGCE, MSc, PhD. Principal Lecturer at the Manchester Metropolitan University, Department of Health Care Studies

Peter Wilkin RMN, CPN, CPT, MA. Primary Mental Health Service manager with Rochdale NHS Trust and a part-time lecturer at the Manchester Metropolitan University, Department of Health Care Studies

Carole Wills RGN, RHV, BSc (Hons.) Health Visitor with Newcastle City Health.

Acknowledgements

The editors and contributors are indebted to those mentors, practitioners, students and colleagues from all specialist practices who over the years have had a significant impact on our understanding of issues that influence teaching and learning in specialist practice.

Specific thanks go to those who contributed through informal research to chapters by Maureen Deacon, Carole Proud and Judith Canham. A special word of thanks goes from Sarah Mattocks to Tina Bishop (Senior Lecturer, Anglia University).

Introduction

Qualified practitioners are responsible and accountable for their own practices. However, the way in which they achieve the skills, knowledge and attributes that enable them to practice with competence and confidence is dependent on how they learnt to be a practitioner. Here, there is no difference between practitioners; whatever the level or length of education, the person who 'teaches' practice has a lasting impact on the neophyte practitioner. Considering the additional responsibilities of specialist community practitioners in nursing and health visiting, very little attention has been paid to the ways in which they are educated in practice. To address this gap, this book is written for practitioners currently undertaking or interested in the mentor role for specialist practitioner students in community settings. Its overall aim is to provide a medium through which mentors can develop their ability to facilitate and meet the learning needs of students in specialist practice. This specialist practice may be nursing, social work or any of the professions allied to medicine, though the focus of the text is on community nursing and health visiting. Even though this text centres on specialist practice, many principles and concepts are transferable to those mentors supporting pre-registration students in community settings.

Whereas all qualified practitioners should have the ability to teach, not all have developed the art of facilitating learning and not all have the academic and practice strengths that will allow them to keep abreast of the demands of specialist practitioner students. The skills and knowledge required of the mentor are vast and include a sound understanding of the complex issues facing the caring professions in the twenty-first century, and the specific educational approaches, strategies and policies that influence learning in practice. The necessary attributes are equally diverse and sometimes contradictory; they hinge on a person who can support and enjoy a student's progress whilst at the same time adopting a critical focus on the professional quality of the student's specialist performance in practice. Through this book we hope that we can enable mentors to have a clearer vision of the contributions they make and the influence they have on practice.

To do justice to the complexity of mentorship we have divided the text into three parts. Part 1, 'The Policy Context', examines the policies and legislation that influence the mentor role. The section starts with an overview of the nature of the specialist practitioner in nursing and health visiting and provides a basic overview of the role and responsibilities of the mentor. Although this is not definitive, it should help readers locate the key elements of their role in the context of the complex concepts and policies that follow. The chapter addressing the policies, strategies and legislation influencing primary care is detailed and here mentors can reflect on their existing knowledge and identify areas for professional development. The review of quality assurance in higher education ends the first section, with a focus on how the quality process may operate, from admission to award. Although at present, mentors may feel detached from the workings of higher education, that is certainly not how the system should operate and we do hope that this and other chapters in Part 1 will inspire, rather than distance, mentors.

Part 2, Theory and Practice Context, explores a wide range of theoretical and practical principles relevant to specialist practice mentorship. Wherever possible we have tried to reduce 'cold theory' (as many other textbooks cover this) and concentrate on more pragmatic issues. In this section you will find examples of how issues are addressed by different people from various academic and work arenas. It might be tempting to question our lack of absolute direction and in our defence we would say that there are a range of possibilities for the application of theory but it is only the unique triumvirate of mentor, student and university teacher who can make the decision as to what is best in a particular situation.

Many of the issues raised in Parts 1 and 2 are revisited in Part 3 'Practice: Opportunities and Challenges', particularly how policy, theory, guidelines and recommendations can be implemented or addressed in practice. Evidence-based practice and research identify the concepts and process of acquiring appropriate evidence and research for practice. Eight chapters then examine each of the current specialist community practices in nursing and health visiting, identifying the uniqueness of the mentor role and trying to solve some of the problems that may confront those facilitating learning and assessing in specialist practice, though often there are no easy answers. Complementing these eight chapters, a specialist practitioner award graduate writes about her experiences as a student and the relationship between her and her mentor. To complete the package a mentor writes about the reality of the role, specifying some of the issues that confront mentors on a regular basis.

It is evident that the role of mentor is not easy when considering the need for ever-increasing knowledge and skills coupled with supportive, facilitative teaching and learning strategies. Rather than providing comfortable solutions to mentorship debates and dilemmas, the penultimate chapter demonstrates why, in the complex health and social care arena, practitioners cannot afford to stand still and ponder but should become active participants in the process of change.

Throughout this book we have, wherever possible, used case studies to illustrate how theories and concepts work in practice. These case studies are based on the real-life experiences of the contributors but have been changed to disguise individuals. We have also used the specialist practice titles in common use in nursing (i.e. health visitor) and not those favoured by the UKCC (1994) and ENB (1995). This is simply a matter of our personal preference.

A word about the term 'mentor'

The publication of a framework to guide educational preparation for mentoring and teaching (ENB & DoH 2001) makes it clear that from September 2001, practitioners who facilitate learning, supervise and assess in *all* pre- and post-registration nursing practice will be 'mentors' prepared for that role. Throughout this book we use the term 'mentor' to describe the person who facilitates learning of specialist practice in community settings.

Judith Canham and Joanne Bennett
June 2001

Part 1
The Policy Context

These first three chapters attempt to provide an overview of policies that have, or should have, a direct impact on the role of the mentor. The first chapter, 'Setting the Scene', focuses on English National Board (ENB) and United Kingdom Central Council (UKCC) policies, standards and frameworks that underpin preparation for specialist community practitioners.

Chapter 2, 'From Policy to Practice', centres its discussion on the considerable practice change that has resulted from Department of Health (DoH) policy, while Chapter 3 is entirely concerned with quality within higher education. Both of these chapters may in the past have been viewed as irrelevant within a 'teaching and learning' text. Our view is that those who provide mentorship for specialist community practitioners need to be up to date with DoH advancements and become more involved with higher education quality processes.

Chapter 1

Setting the Scene: Concepts of Specialist Practitioner and Specialist Practice Mentor

Judith Canham

Before embarking on a journey through the policies that influence both the mentor and what is to be learnt by the specialist practitioner student, this chapter provides an overview of the concepts of specialist practitioner and mentor. Visualising the expectations of specialist practitioners in conjunction with your role as mentor should identify why we place so much importance on policy and theory early on in the text.

Specialist practice

There is a difference between the nurse who works in a specialist practice and a specialist practitioner (UKCC 1994). Although many of the former may have achieved the skills, knowledge and attributes of the specialist practitioner through years of experience and personal study, there is no guarantee that this transition will have occurred. Specific education and assessment is the way in which the public, employers, colleagues and professional bodies can be assured that a practitioner has successfully completed the theoretical and practice elements of an educational programme designed to meet specialist practitioner outcomes. The UKCC (1994) and ENB (1995) clearly define specialist practice in exactly the same way:

> 'Whilst pre-registration education provides practitioners with the knowledge, skills and attributes to give safe and effective care, this alone does not prepare them adequately to meet additional specialist needs. Specialist health care and specialist patient/client requirements call for additional education for safe and effective practice. There is, therefore, a need for *some* practitioners to *exercise higher levels of judgement and discretion* in clinical care in order to function as specialist practitioners. Such specialist practitioners should be able to demonstrate *higher levels of clinical decision making and will be able to monitor and improve standards of care through supervision of practice, clinical audit, the provision of skilled professional leadership and the devel-*

3

*opment of practice through research, teaching and the support of profes-
sional colleagues.'* (my italics)

(UKCC 1994, p. 9 and ENB 1995, p. 22)

Translating this definition of the specialist practitioner into education and
practice is possible through a series of standards for specialist education and
practice (ENB 1995 pp. 22–8). For example the practitioner should:

'Lead and clinically direct the professional team to ensure the implementation and monitoring of quality assured standards of care by effective
and efficient management of finite resources.'

(ENB 1995, 18.10, p. 23)

The ENB (1995) standard statements clarify the specific ways in which the
specialist practitioner is different from a nurse who works in that practice, and
thus the learning needs of specialist students. From these standards, teachers
and mentors are able to identify aims and learning outcomes for facilitating
learning, teaching and assessing in both theory and practice.

At the end of their course of education, all specialist practitioners need to be
able to articulate, justify and defend current and projected practices in light of
both health policy and rhetoric. It is essential that in nursing and health visiting
a specialist community practitioner should be capable of leading practice
pivotal to the health, care and well-being of the UK population.

Programme organisation to meet specialist practitioner outcomes

Programmes leading to a Specialist Practitioner Award must focus on four
main areas (UKCC 1994, 1998; ENB 1995) that will enable students to meet the
demands of specialist practice and the specialist practitioner role:

- **Clinical nursing practice** provides students with opportunities to
  acquire the knowledge and skills necessary to meet the specialist clinical
  needs of patients/clients.
- **Care and programme management** addresses the needs of individual
  patients, the family, the community and the environment of care through
  preparing the student to draw together the necessary agencies, professionals and non-professionals to meet identified need. The focus includes
  health promotion and skilled intervention.
- **Clinical practice development** addresses issues such as standard setting and quality assurance as well as practice development and research
  relating to the specialist area.
- **Clinical practice leadership** prepares students to lead and deliver
  services that are sensitive to consumer need as well as enabling them
  to support and teach other professional colleagues and students in
  practice.

Although educational programmes in nursing and health visiting have to adhere to ENB direction, the precise way in which courses are organised varies. The most important point for mentors is that all specialist practitioner courses must be divided equally between theory and practice: a 50/50 split. This means that in a course of 34 weeks, the specialist student will be spending 17 weeks in placement with a mentor.

Additionally, education for specialist practitioners must consist of a common core of no less than one third and no more than two thirds of the entire course (ENB 1995). The specific specialist practice element is no less than one third of the course, allowing students to focus on their future practice but not to the detriment of issues common to all students. (In reality students spend far more than one third of the course addressing specialist issues as they relate core material to specialist practice in all written and practice assessments.) The division of learning time benefits students by giving them both a broad and a specific education that prepares them for a professional career demanding a wide knowledge base and a collaborative working style.

The academic level of preparation for specialist practice

In 1994 the UKCC determined that pre-registration nurse education was to be at a minimum of diploma level and that specialist practitioner (post-registration) education would be at a minimum of degree level (academic level III) by virtue of natural progression. At the time of writing (2001) most specialist practitioner applicants are eligible to enter level III, having already completed pre-registration nurse education with a Diploma of Higher Education (Nursing) or, having undertaken post-registration level II/Diploma of Higher Education studies. Most higher education institutes (HEIs) have additional entry criteria that ask for evidence of specific study and relevant experience before students will be admitted to the programme. These entry criteria are to ensure that students entering degree studies are professionally ready and academically able to undertake the programme.

The thinking behind the 1994 change to pre-registration nursing and specialist practitioner education (UKCC 1994) was centred on the health needs of the population and the needs of the health services in the twenty-first century. However, aside from 'natural progression' there appears to have been little evidence to support the move of specialist practice to degree level. Whether or not specialist practice makes a real difference to practice by being at degree level has yet to be seen, though experience suggests that most students utilise the critical skills of degree education in their theoretical and practical work. (For detail of critical skills see Chapter 4.)

Professional and organisational influence on preparation for specialist practice

In relation to present educational policy, it is interesting that despite the implication that specialist practice builds on and develops existing skills, neither the UKCC (1994) nor ENB (1995) clarify the period or place within which these existing skills should have been consolidated. Because of this fudging, employment issues and professional preferences have been able to supersede the purpose of education, with students entering specialist practitioner programmes at different levels of preparedness. The prime example is health visiting where very few students have previously worked in that setting, as health visiting has steadfastly opposed a skill mix and, ironically, suffers a chronic staff shortage. Thus some students have to travel further and faster along the role preparation continuum than others. Although it could be suggested that health visitor students have less to unlearn or that they use the concept and argument of 'Life Long Learning' (ENB 1995) to balance the anomaly, this does not alter the fact that on qualification, a health visitor with a minimum of 32 weeks education and experience will be a specialist practitioner expected by the public to possess all the skills, knowledge and attributes of the role. This situation would simply not occur within (for example) intensive care units where a nurse undertaking the ENB 100 is likely to have been working within the speciality before embarking on the course and will not expect to lead practice immediately after qualification.

Despite the principle that post-registration education should be linked to service need, many specialist practitioner students find themselves in a restricting grade on qualification. (In a few cases, qualifying students are not employed by their sponsoring authority.) This means that at the end of their course some students may be constrained in their ability to apply and consolidate learning in practice. Interestingly this rarely applies to health visiting graduates who are invariably employed as specialist practitioners, but it frequently applies to district nurse graduates who often have considerable pre-course experience. Mentors need to be clear that all specialist students need to learn and develop their specialist practitioner competencies to the same level, despite their future career possibilities. However, an unclear future can have considerable impact on students' motivation during the course especially as it draws to an end, and there is no easy way to counter apathy or anger directed at employment strategies.

The mentor for specialist practice in community settings

While specialist practice has developed since the publication of *The Future of Professional Practice* (UKCC 1994), the role of the mentor for specialist community practice has yet to be determined adequately by either the ENB or UKCC, pre-registration practice being the priority within policy (ENB & DoH 2001). Prevarication in policy direction between 1994 and 2001 meant that HEIs set their own standards for mentors of specialist practitioner courses. By and large these HEI standards worked well and met the learning needs of specialist students, the continuing professional development needs of mentors and quality management within service.

Preparation of mentors and teachers: a new framework for guidance (ENB & DoH 2001)

The term mentor is used to denote the role of the nurse, midwife or health visitor who facilitates learning and assesses students in the practice setting (ENB & DoH 2001, p. 6). The mentor role will be to:

- Facilitate learning across pre- and *post-registration programmes* (my italics)
- Supervise, support and guide students in practice in institutions and non-institutional settings
- Implement approved assessed procedures.

(ENB & DoH 2001, p. 9)

Interestingly, the ENB fails to clarify any real difference between the needs of a pre-registration student and the needs of a specialist practitioner student required to develop their first level skills in a specific practice.

The role of the 'new' practice educator (ENB & DoH 2001) denotes a role focused on:

- Learning in the practice setting
- The management of resources and student experiences
- Providing support and guidance to mentors and other service personnel who contribute to the student's experience in practice.

(ENB & DoH, p. 15)

The ENB and DoH (2001) framework may have confounded clarity of title (once again) but we can be confident that issues of fundamental importance to mentors in community settings are relatively constant. Of significant interest is that research about the role of the mentor (by whatever name) within post-registration community education is scant (Maggs & Purr 1989; Canham 1991). The dearth of empirical study has resulted in guiding policy, theory and texts being based predominantly on practice placements and teachers of pre-registration students, mainly in institutional settings. Later in this book you will find that many contributors working directly with mentors and specialist students have undertaken small scale studies that add to the knowledge base.

Historical perspectives

Only district nursing and health visiting have a strong history of mentoring (practice teaching) where mentors were respectively known as practical work teachers and field work teachers until 1989 when joint training for the role changed the role title to community practice teachers (CPTs). Other community practices, such as general practice nursing, had long recognised the need for a specific practice mentor but were often thwarted by lack of support from their employers.

Although in many cases 'sitting with Nellie' would have been the main way of learning how to be a school nurse, for example, in some practices even this elementary technique was ignored as the following case study illustrates.

'When I was doing my community practice nurse (CPN) training back in 1980, it was all so different from how CPN [community mental health nurse] students are educated today. I was already working as a CPN before I went on the course at Manchester Poly. You'd probably say I was an unqualified CPN, but we didn't really note the difference. While I was doing the course I still managed a case load and there was no one specific to support me. Occasionally my manager would ask how I was getting on but I think he was more interested in getting me back to full-time work.

The course was interesting and I know I learned a lot, but here's the rub, in practice I was just left to my own devices. Well I'd been doing the job hadn't I so who was going to question me? I did the essays for the Poly and my manager signed my practice assessment form, but no one, absolutely no one questioned my existing practice or my skills with clients. I don't think my practice changed much during the course and it was only when I got into clinical supervision and started questioning myself, that I realised there were real problems with my practice. Not major, I wasn't going to kill anybody, but, well to be honest, I was still functioning in an institutional style. My practice was still based on a closed ward, I didn't lead, I didn't teach and I certainly didn't get myself involved in practice development.

When I first took on this role [mentor] my student had been a G grade colleague and presumed that he'd just carry on. It was hard at first as we challenged each other's role but eventually I just told him that he had to show me that he was able to be a specialist practitioner not just another mental health nurse working in the community. We worked through the ENB stuff [Life Long Learners] and eventually both of us could see a real difference in his practice. He's probably more of a clinical leader than me now but I suppose that's just part of the role, isn't it?'

Case Study 1.1 Moving toward good mentorship

Aside from health visiting, and to some extent district nursing, it was common practice to be employed as an unqualified community nurse, and training procedures were simply a method of securing a better grade or utilising training monies. In such cases, the old system of training may have done little more than ensure that custom and practice were continued.

Although the difference between the past and current education for specialist practitioners should be stark, where there is no mandatory requirement for the specialist practitioner qualification, secondment and sponsorship may still be a matter of using up monies for education, whilst applying natural progression in practice. Practice that legitimises promotion without appropriate education suggests that education is not fundamental to the development of practitioners or practice and that when specialist education is utilised, it is without wholehearted recognition of its potential to enable a different and special practitioner. Unfortunately the ENB and DoH framework (2001) does little to support education in practice for specialist students. Despite policy direction, or the lack of it, there should be little doubt that unless both the mentor and specialist practitioner student are aware of the purpose of education, the practice placement will be simply a matter of marking time rather than using the opportunity productively.

The role of the mentor

Regardless of the new framework (ENB & DoH 2001) mentors are instrumental in ensuring that newly qualified specialist practitioners are competent at all aspects of a dynamic role. The complexity of the role of mentor is heightened by its dual nature; it is not a joint role where part of the time is given over to teaching and part to practice – both parts of the role are carried out simultaneously (Wong & Wong 1987; Canham 1991). As existing mentors know, this is no easy task when considering the demands of ill or distressed patients/clients and carers, and challenging students. A study of pre- and post-registration mentors (Davies *et al.* 1995) identified that issues such as the time to undertake the role properly were of great concern. Within specialist practice, the student and mentor will experience an intense relationship for the duration of the course and the lack of professional space within this unity demands consideration vis-à-vis its potential impact on both student and mentor. For example, the mentor may need to utilise the resources offered by other practitioners, have a strategy for creating some emotional and physical space, have given thought to managing a 'tense' student-mentor relationship and, when the time is right, have the confidence to allow the student professional freedom.

Although a unique strength of the mentor should be undisputed clinical expertise, that by itself is insufficient to ensure that the standard of practice learning is developed or maintained at the level expected by the public and the NHS. Davies *et al.* (1995) noted that three-quarters of mentors were not undertaking continuing professional development and very few had undertaken diploma or degree studies, perhaps having shelved their academic study to concentrate on practice issues. Davies *et al.* (1995) also found that most mentors were unable to articulate why they did what they did. In other words they were unable to justify the basis of their teaching, facilitating and assessing. As one of the benefits of degree study for specialist students is the development of critical thinking, mentors need similar study to equip themselves not only for facilitating student development, but also for the ability to do as students do: defend decisions and articulate practice.

Uncovering specialist practice

The role-modelling aspect of the mentoring role cannot be disputed (Jarvis & Gibson 1997) especially when the placement is continuous. However if the role model lacks the requisite skills, knowledge and attributes, there are two possible outcomes. Either the student will not recognise the deficiency and will learn an incomplete role, or the student will identify the deficiency and become frustrated with the mentor. Experience of specialist students suggests that students' relationships with mentors depend partly on mentors' deep and critical understanding of practice and thus, as can be seen in case study 1.2, the mentor's ability to assist learning of obscure and challenging concepts.

'My very first visit in practice was a 'crisis call' to the family of a woman who'd just died. She had looked after her middle-aged son with Down's syndrome. When we [student and mentor] got to the house, the family were really abusive, throwing insults at both of us and the whole NHS. I would have walked away but somehow Fozia calmed them down and oh, less than an hour later we left the house, having managed all their concerns. I know this sounds daft but I thought the way she handled the situation was mysterious.

Afterwards, Fozia made me stand in her proverbial shoes and look at the whole incident in detail. When they came to the door shouting, she immediately changed her physical stance, became quiet and serious and maintained good but not staring eye contact. She had also moved herself to stand slightly in front of me; I didn't realise this at the time. While she was doing this and listening she was also thinking 'why are they angry, will seeing two people at the door make things worse, what are their expectations of the NHS and the LD [learning disability] service, how may we have failed them, what care options are available, what theories are relevant here?' and so on.

Anyway the point of all this is that she didn't fob me off with 'oh you'll learn with experience', she knew exactly what she'd done and why. Now that was really impressive. Do you know that we spent the whole afternoon discussing that situation. I suppose care is only mysterious when you don't know why it happens.'

Case Study 1.2 Uncovering the mysteries of specialist practice

Context

Community care has changed substantially over the past ten years. Care and treatments have changed and the public has very different expectations of the caring professions. In most cases there are fewer staff to manage more complex cases and the demands on practitioners from all sides are enormous. Although there is substantial policy to guide the education of specialist practitioner students who will lead and develop practice, this means very little without a mentor capable of facilitating appropriate learning through, for and in practice. It is often said that the role of, for example, the health visitor or school health nurse is pivotal to quality health and health care. I would argue that in reality, this defining role belongs to mentors. Without their expertise, the likelihood is that practice will remain static with few creative care ideas and little practice development. Mentors have the opportunity to enable the next generation of specialist practitioners to develop the knowledge, skills and attributes that will have a fundamental impact on care provision.

Chapter 2
From Policy to Practice

Joanne Bennett

This chapter considers the ways in which health and health care have been subject to rapid change, specifically since 1997. Government health policy dictates both the way in which health services are organised and the roles of all practitioners working within these services. These policies are of significant interest to mentors in that not only will mentors be at the forefront of change as practitioners but they will also be the guiding lights for specialist practitioner students for whom 'change' and 'new' policies will be a way of life.

Joanne Bennett uses this chapter to try and make complex policy intelligible. She clearly identifies both the salient points and the challenges that lie ahead for students and mentors.

Introduction

The organisation, management and delivery of health care in the UK are all undergoing change at an unprecedented rate. The New Labour Government is committed to modernising the NHS and has proposed a 'third way' of working so that quality is at the forefront of service delivery, which in turn is based on partnership and is organised and integrated around patient needs. Furthermore, the Government is committed to tackling the causes of ill health as well as providing fast and effective treatment for those with an established illness or disability. Nowhere are these changes more evident than in the delivery of primary health care. The reconstruction of the agenda is fast, with the first wave of Primary Care Groups (PCGs) established in April 1999 and the first Primary Care Trusts (PCTs) in April 2000.

Change does not operate in a vacuum and the effects of changes in policy have had, and indeed continue to have, a considerable impact on the roles, responsibilities and boundaries of those practitioners involved in the organisation, management and delivery of services in primary care. In order to effectively respond to and implement the Government's agenda, professionals need to be well informed and prepared to change and develop services. One way of addressing this is through appropriate education for and in practice. It must however be acknowledged that this in itself is insufficient to guarantee that the goals of policy will be transferred into action. The world of practice is far too complex, fragmented and fluid to attempt to find all of the solutions through preparation for specialist practice. It is a process which requires unprecedented levels of trust and co-operation across agencies, which cannot be achieved through education alone.

In acknowledging this, I am also acknowledging the limited scope of this chapter, which primarily focuses on the implications of a fairly narrow area of health policy for the preparation of specialist practitioners. I will begin by briefly outlining some of the policy changes that have influenced primary health care delivery in general, before focusing on primary health care nursing more specifically since the introduction of market mechanisms in the 1990s. Difficulties inherent within this system will be discussed in the context of the Labour Government's agenda which was outlined in the white paper, *The New NHS Modern and Dependable* (DoH 1997a), *Saving Lives – Our Healthier Nation* (DoH 1999b) and *The NHS Plan* (DoH 2000a). Many of the policy issues raised in this chapter will be revisited and further developed in subsequent chapters.

The need for change

The structure of the British welfare state in areas of health and social policy were basically the same in 1987 as they had been in 1979, with the state both funding and providing services to the vast majority of the population. However, the 1980s witnessed a decade of Thatcherism, and it was in this period that we witnessed major challenges to the basic structure of the welfare state on the grounds that it was too bureaucratic and that the professions were based on self-interest, inefficiency and ineffectiveness (Le Grand 1990; Wilding 1992). Thatcherism further asserted the need to encourage citizens to accept responsibility and obligation in areas of welfare policy.

The New Right sought to address such issues by introducing competition into the area of health care provision through the introduction of active market mechanisms and the development of an internal market. This was the main objective of the white paper *Working for Patients* (DoH 1989a). The implementation of General Practitioner Fundholding (GPFH) in April 1991 (DoH 1989a) witnessed the start of the introduction of market mechanisms into general practice settings. GP fundholders were delegated purchasing functions for a limited range of services which, in the early days, included some hospital services, practice staff and drugs. This was later extended to include community nursing, dietetics and chiropody. The bulk of the social care reforms were deferred until 1 April 1993, when we saw the implementation of the community care part of the NHS and Community Care Act 1990. This incorporated the main recommendations of the white paper, *Caring for People* (DoH 1989b) and brought with it the strengthening of a mixed economy of care in this area.

A number of criticisms emerged from this system which led the newly elected Labour Government to outline changes to the organisation and delivery of health care evident in *The New NHS Modern and Dependable* (DoH 1997a), *Saving Lives – Our Healthier Nation* (DoH 1999b) and more recently, *The NHS Plan* (DoH 2000a). For example, in *The New NHS Modern and Dependable* (DoH 1997a) it was argued that the development of the internal market and the bureaucracy created through the development of this system did little to tackle issues of integration across health and social care. This was particularly evident when a service user had multiple needs. The Government therefore sought to eradicate the bureaucracy created by this system through reducing the number of commissioning bodies from 3600 to as few as 500 with the redirection of savings from reduced administrative costs to patient care. These problems had arguably been exacerbated by the short-term nature of the contracts that had evolved through the internal market, which had led to instability in the market as well as increased administrative costs. Under the new arrangements it was proposed that the length of a contract should be increased to a minimum of three years.

Furthermore, the Government wanted to eradicate popular perceptions of GPFH whereby it was proposed that a two-tiered system had been created and that some doctors were in a stronger position to negotiate a better deal for patients, based on finance rather than clinical reasoning. Indeed, quality of service provision was a concern within the NHS where considerable variations in quality were observed. Even where good practice was evident the Government noted that there was a reluctance to share this because of the competition created by the internal market. The Government's vision for the National Health Service was therefore based on the development of a quality service organised and integrated around patient needs that tackled the causes of ill health, as well as illness and disability. The proposal was to replace the internal market with a system of integrated care (DoH 1997a). The means of achieving this was through the framework of clinical governance and health improvement programmes (HImPs); Primary Care Groups and Primary Care Trusts were the vehicle for realising this within primary health care. The process was also aided through the removal of legal obstacles to joint working which are evident in the partnership flexibility's section of the 1999 Health Act.

The development of primary care groups

The development of Primary Care Groups (PCGs) was the Government's response to dealing with some of the concerns outlined above. PCGs typically serve around 100 000 patients and are developed around natural communities. Through bringing groups of GPs and community nurses in each area together, and giving them responsibility for commissioning services for local patients, it is envisaged that there will be increased efficiency and quality for the patient. PCGs may choose to operate at one of four levels, which range from that of acting in an advisory capacity to the Health Authority to accepting devolved operation and management. A board that acts as a subcommittee to the Health Authority governs each PCG. Representation on the board should include:

- General Practitioners   4–7
- Community nurses/practice nurses   1–2

- Social services representative   1
- Lay representative   1
- Health Authority non-executive member   1
- Chief   1

Opportunities have subsequently been made available for the development of care trusts. Under this arrangement a single multi-purpose body would be responsible for all health and social care.

The development of PCGs and the representation of nurses at board level are a significant move forward for nursing in that nurses have been provided with an opportunity to voice their views and share their knowledge and expertise. However, for the majority of nurses this means developing new skills such as those required for marketing and commissioning. Perhaps even more challenging is the need to overcome the power differential that has existed, and in many areas continues to exist, between the medical profession and nursing. Prior to teasing out some of the implications of these changes on the role and preparation of the community specialist practitioner, it is important to consider briefly the role and functions of PCGs.

Function of Primary Care Groups (PCGs)

Primary Care Groups are seen as an essential part of the modernisation process and are charged with a number of functions:

- Improving the health of their community
- Developing primary care and community services across the PCG
- Advising on, or commissioning directly, a range of hospital services to meet patient needs.

Improving the health of the community

Primary Care Groups are charged with improving the health of the community through:

(1) Identifying the health needs of the community
(2) Informing and contributing to the local health improvement programme
(3) Working with other agencies (e.g. social services and other local government agencies) to ensure the co-ordination and integration of service delivery
(4) Involving the public to ensure the appropriateness of services.

(DoH 1998c)

Health Improvement Programmes (HImPs) are seen as the local strategy for improving health and healthcare (DoH 1998d). They are viewed as the mechanism to deliver national targets in each Health Authority area. It is the Health Authority that has the lead responsibility for drawing up the HImP in consultation with NHS Trusts, PCGs, other primary care professionals such as

15

dentists, opticians and pharmacists, the public and partner organisations (DoH 1997a).

Indeed, the green paper, *Our Healthier Nation* (DoH 1999b) identified how PCGs would be responsible for contributing to and implementing HImPs which reflect local perspectives and are delivered in partnership with key local organisations. The process for developing the HImP sets out to bring together the NHS, local authorities and others to develop a strategic framework for improving health, tackling inequality and developing a faster service with high standards (DoH 1998d). Primary Care Groups are seen to be closest to the population and as such they are able to draw on their local knowledge to assist in the process of identifying health need as well as providing a direct response to community health problems. For example, they may work with local schools to reduce smoking or drug use, or they may use a community development approach to improve the health of those who have difficulty accessing health care facilities. This will require a shift in both thinking and practice for the majority of community nurses who tend to work with staff from their own specialist area of community nursing to develop health profiles.

Developing primary care and community services across the Primary Care Group

The second area of responsibility allocated to PCGs is the development of primary care and community services across their area through:

(1) Developing and supporting primary and community provision
(2) Reducing variation in the provision of services
(3) Improving the quality and standards of provision through the framework of clinical governance
(4) Integrating the delivery of primary and community health services.

(DoH 1998c)

The development of high quality services in primary and community care is dependent on the promotion of best practice. It is envisaged that in time clinical governance will provide the framework for identifying good practice and also those areas which need to improve. In order to realise its goal and encourage the sharing of information about care, clinical governance must be carried out in an atmosphere of trust and support and involve all professionals and partners in care delivery. The process is to be aided through the development of national service frameworks in key areas and the mandatory use of partnership flexibilities.

The Health Service Circular (DoH 1998e) highlights the ten points of clinical governance from *The New NHS*, which are about:

● Quality improvement processes such as clinical audit being in place
● Leadership skills being developed at a clinical team level
● Evidence-based practice being in day-to-day use with an infrastructure to support it

- Good practice and innovations which have been evaluated being systematically disseminated both within the organisation and externally
- Clinical risk reduction programmes being in place
- Adverse events being openly investigated and learned from
- Lessons for clinical practice being learned from the input of patients
- Poor clinical practice being recognised at an early stage and dealt with to prevent harm to patients and to improve practitioners' performance
- The principles of clinical governance being reflected in all professional development programmes
- The quality of data gathered to monitor clinical care being of a high standard.

To ensure that this agenda is taken forward, each PCG must appoint a senior health professional to take clinical governance forward. This may or may not be the same person identified as taking a lead for education and training. However, all staff functioning at a specialist practitioner level must develop knowledge, understanding and skills in research (see Chapter 9), practice development, quality assurance, leadership and managing change, risk management and health needs analysis.

Advise on, or commission directly, a range of hospital services to meet patient need

Finally, PCGs are responsible for advising on, or commissioning directly, a range of hospital services to meet patient needs by:

(1) Commissioning high quality services
(2) Monitoring the performance of providers against service agreements
(3) Contributing to the national drive to reduce waiting lists.

(Adapted from DoH 1998c)

Due to the instability which resulted from short-term contracts in the internal market the government set out new arrangements for commissioning services which covered:

- The ending of annual contracts and the introduction of NHS service agreements
- The development of long-term service agreements
- More effective arrangements for the commissioning of specialist services
- The ending of extra contractual referrals

(DoH 1998f)

There is also the expectation that the responsibility for commissioning will be delegated from the Health Authorities to PCGs and PCTs. For some this means developing new areas of expertise.

Implications for the preparation of specialist practitioners and the role of the mentor

The meaningful contribution of the specialist practitioner is crucial to the successful implementation of these reforms. This will invariably mean that routines and procedures that have been developed over many years to cope with the complexity of practice in community nursing must be explored and challenged. In many areas these routines have been developed to deal with large case-loads which have often been combined with inadequate resources (and/or inappropriately used resources), conflicting goals and organisational demands. Some professionals have also used them in an attempt to maintain their identity and professional autonomy. These practices must be uncovered and explored in a way that attempts to capitalise on the potential of this group. Moves forward can only be achieved if sufficient attention is paid to both the initial preparation of community specialist practitioners and the continuing professional development of all staff working within the arena of primary care.

Exploration of policy in this area clearly indicates that the specialist practitioner must demonstrate that they are able to work in partnership with others to:

- Identify and explore strategies to meet the health needs of the local population
- Address the public health agenda – this must be approached from the perspective of both the individual and the community
- Develop approaches to integrated care, chronic disease management and intermediate care
- Develop nurse-led services
- Critically review existing service delivery and skill mix and develop integrated approaches to meeting need, e.g. rapid response teams to meet intermediate care needs
- Strengthen the contribution of service users so that they play a stronger role in the shaping and evaluation of services
- Operate within the framework of clinical governance, demonstrating evidence-based practice which is delivered within national frameworks (see Chapter 9); the ability to monitor quality is central to this process
- Engage in research and/or practice development
- Understand the nurses' role/potential role in the commissioning of services
- Identify and plan to meet education and training needs of nursing team linked to needs of primary health care team and the organisation
- Demonstrate the ability to work with others to lead and change practice.

Indeed, many of these requirements are mirrored in the characteristics of the specialist practitioner (UKCC 1994, 1998b). Although there have been considerable changes to the standard, kind and content of specialist practitioner courses, recent Government policy has reinforced the need for their continual development to meet the challenges of primary care provision and the public health agenda. Furthermore, service evaluation in some areas of practice (Audit Commission 1999) and the recent strategy for nursing outlined in *Making a Difference* (DoH 1999a) have stated the need to review current practice particularly in areas such as initiating and managing change, practice, development, public health and chronic disease management as well as explore opportunities for new ways of working, for example nurse-led services.

Progression is arguably dependent on the development of visionary leaders who can work across professional and organisational boundaries to inspire and motivate teams to work together to meet the health needs of the population. The extent to which current specialist practitioner preparation equips nurses for this role is debatable, as is the assumption that all community nurses have the necessary requirements to fulfil this role. Furthermore, while all specialist practitioner courses must meet ENB requirements, the way in which they are met varies between higher education institutions and between routes within the same institution depending on the area of preparation being undertaken. In addition to this, the teaching and learning approaches adopted in both university settings and practice clearly impact on the extent to which these practitioners are fit for contemporary practice. In turn, these approaches are further influenced by the infrastructure of both environments.

Despite such variations, it is clearly no longer acceptable to explore theoretical debates underpinning practice in isolation from practical experience and competency development. It must be done in a way that demonstrates that the practitioner is able to provide a quality service which is organised and integrated around patient/service user need. For example, the majority of specialist practitioner courses require students to draw on the knowledge gained through classroom debate as well as from the experiences and the local knowledge of their mentors, to undertake a health needs assessment and analysis of the local population. Due to time constraints and traditional ways of working, it is not uncommon for this work to be undertaken in isolation from other practitioners working in the area, with separate profiles for district nurses and health visitors being found on the same office shelf. Furthermore, strategies have yet to be developed to feed this information to local PCGs and PCTs and to strengthen the voice of community nurses in the commissioning of services. There is therefore a need for the course team (which includes staff from higher education and practice) to develop strategies which encourage students to work with others in the practice setting to develop a more integrated approach to undertaking a health needs analysis, which in turn encourages the development of partnerships and cross-organisational working as well as assisting nurses to develop skills in marketing and commissioning. At present not all specialist practitioner students are required to do this.

Similarly, the student's exposure to public health has been limited. While students may engage in debates in the classroom which encompass a variety of approaches to public health, the majority of their experiences in practice centre on the needs of the individual rather than the community or population. Again, the challenge for all those involved in the preparation of specialist practitioners is to explore and further develop strategies which encourage and expose students to new ways of working focusing on population health and community development, not just the needs of individuals and families. In doing so, the student will be exposed to the reality of developing alliances and partnerships between professions and across agencies in the public, voluntary and independent sectors. Implicit within this is the need to develop strategies to involve service users in this process.

Graduates from specialist practitioner courses must also have demonstrated how they are able to lead a team to develop practice. It is no longer acceptable for students to explore theoretical debates around change, practice development and the development of evidence-based practice (to name but a few) without providing evidence to demonstrate how they have used this knowledge in practice. In doing so they will need to work with a team to develop an area of practice based on an identified need. This will involve skills in research appreciation, leadership, teamwork, networking and evaluation.

Summary

These are but a few of the challenges that lie ahead for all those involved in the preparation of specialist practitioners. I have clearly only touched on the implications of a fairly limited area of health policy, which is subject to continual change, on the role and preparation of the specialist practitioner. The following chapters will endeavour to outline some of the strategies currently in use to prepare these practitioners for the ever-changing world of practice, together with some of the strengths and limitations of these approaches.

Chapter 3

Maintaining and Developing Quality and Equity within Higher Education Programmes

Mary Dunning

As the mentors of specialist community practitioner students facilitate half of the students' educational preparation, it follows that mentors should be involved in HEI policy. In this chapter Mary Dunning provides detail of the quality process at one HEI, starting with how courses of education are validated and moving through to the continual assurance of quality educational provision. Although the policies within this chapter are specific to one HEI, the principles will be common to all those HEIs that mentors work with.

It is our hope that mentors will be motivated to become involved in the development and maintenance of HEI quality by contributing to validation, on-going assurance, review and audit quality enhancement.

Introduction

The purpose of this chapter is to provide an overview of how quality is maintained within higher education institutions (HEIs). This is particularly important given that HEIs are largely self-regulating and therefore responsible for ensuring and demonstrating rigour in safeguarding standards for the teaching, learning and assessment of their programmes and awards. This responsibility is discharged in a context of national and internal systems of quality assurance, audit and enhancement. Most quality assurance systems have a set of underlying values such as Maxwell's (1984) principles of equity, effectiveness, appropriateness, accessibility, responsiveness and humanity. These underpinning values should be transparent and evident within quality systems in HEIs.

HEIs are accountable to a variety of stakeholders for the quality of their provision: to the students, employers, the public and themselves. In the context of professional activity they are also accountable to professional statutory bodies (e.g. English National Board (ENB)), commissioners (e.g. workforce development confederations), partners who provide workplace experience and users of the service. The importance that HEIs place on quality can be seen in their mission statements. For example, at the University of Northumbria at Newcastle (UNN) the mission statement states that the university is characterised by 'the outstanding quality of teaching and research' (UNN 1999a). Embedded in further statements are the values of the organisation in access, equity, cost-effectiveness, responsiveness to students and employers and development of the full human potential of its students. Stakeholders are able to judge provision against the mission and the stated value.

Key quality systems

The following elements should be present both within the institution and in the systems used by external bodies to scrutinise HEIs in relation to the quality of their provision.

Quality assurance: The strategies, systems, processes and policies by which an institution assures itself and others of the quality and standards of its provision.
Quality audit: A system of checking that its quality assurance systems are in place and functioning.
Quality management and control: The managerial systems, structures and roles that the organisation adapts in order that the quality assurance processes are implemented. Quality control is where the locus of responsibility lies within these systems.
Quality enhancement: The strategies, plans, tactics and mechanisms by which an institution ensures that the quality of its provision is improved.

Quality assurance

Everyone who works within a university or is a partner in providing learning for students has a responsibility to ensure the quality of the programmes. This tenet should be embedded within the academic culture of the university, and quality systems should be owned by all concerned.

The validation process

The course will be designed by a group of experts within the field, internal and external to the university. The curriculum planning team will need to know the latest knowledge and practices within the discipline in order to inform the curriculum content. The aims and outcomes that the students will achieve and how they are assessed, learning and teaching methodologies, academic level and credit and the organisation of the delivery, all need to be clearly stated. The university regulations on how students progress through the course and what support and guidance they receive need to be incorporated into the curriculum document. Learning resources to support the students' learning and the quality assurance and management systems in the programme need to be identified. The team also has to ensure ENB standards and regulations are included. This results in a definitive course document that enables the student and others to know the intentions and outcomes of the course.

Critical scrutiny of this new course will take place at a validation event. A team of managers, practitioners and peers from within the university, inter and intra to the discipline, external experts and ENB approved external examiners will question the course team about their intent. This peer evaluation assures that the course is of a standard for the award of the university, for professional practice and for the purpose of the intended employment.

On-going assurance

Once the community specialist practitioner course is approved for five-year periods, HEIs continue to quality assure the programme using the following:

- Annual review
- External examining
- Curriculum change

Annual review

The course will be managed by a Programme Director (a senior academic) and a Programme Management Group which has responsibility to manage the student's experience and to ensure the standard and quality of delivery. The group should have representation from teachers, students, mentors and if possible users of the service.

Annual academic quality review (AAQR) takes place both for the course and the subject area and includes formal feedback from the students, contributing teachers, mentors and external examiners. This review analyses the qualitative data from evaluations plus the quantitative data from student entry, progression and exit statistics. The review identifies areas of strength and possible areas for development, actions with target dates and named responsible person(s). It should refer back to and report on the previous year's review and actions. Feedback should be given to students and other stakeholders on the actions achieved and to be taken; it is in this way that 'quality loops' are formed. Quality review can therefore be seen as a continuous process.

External examiners

The role of external examiners is key to the quality assurance systems of British higher education. All courses must have scrutiny by an independent expert in the discipline. External examiners are appointed by the university, usually for a period of three to five years, against a set of criteria that includes experience and knowledge. Any close links that are already in existence with the university are also identified. The external examiner will also need to be approved by the ENB.

External examiners have the following key purposes:

- To assist in the comparison of academic standards across the awards and units of the university curriculum
- To verify that the standards set are appropriate for the awards and units of the university and that such standards are assured
- To ensure that the assessment process is fair and is fairly operated in the marking, grading and classification of student performance.

(UNN 1999b)

In order to perform their task external examiners need to be familiar with university rules and regulations for assessment as well as the definitive course document. They scutinise a representative selection of student work and attend Examination Boards. In the case of this course they also need to scutinise practice assessments, by talking to mentors and students and by examining practice assessment documentation.

A formal report is submitted each year from the external examiner, which informs the AAQR. The programme team should respond to this report in writing. Good practice in many HEIs is also to have external examiner reports analysed by academics not directly involved in the course in order to identify cross-programme issues. At UNN members of the faculty quality committee do this.

Curriculum change

All courses will be subject to change during the time of their approval. This change is the result of evaluations from the student, external examiner and other stakeholders, as well as new research findings and in the case of this course, policy change in the NHS. It is important that change can occur, often quickly; however it is also important that changes are subject to quality assurance processes. Universities are often criticised that they are very slow in coping with change. Many have listened to this criticism and are exploring ways that on-going change can be quality assured quickly at the closest point to delivery. This is often achieved by devolving responsibility to school or division level.

External review

The processes described so far are internal to the university. Universities are also subject to external scrutiny. There are three other bodies that have a formal role in the quality assurance of the course. They are:

- The Quality Assurance Agency (QAA)
- The professional and statutory body (National Boards for Nursing, Midwifery and Health Visiting)
- The commissioner (workforce development confederations).

The Quality Assurance Agency

The Quality Assurance Agency (QAA) was established in 1997 as an independent body to provide an integrated quality assurance service for UK higher education institutions. The Agency's mission is 'to promote public confidence that the quality of provision and the standard of awards in higher education are being safeguarded and enhanced'. Its core business is to review the quality and standards of higher education in universities and colleges. It does this by auditing institutional arrangements for managing quality and standards including arrangements for collaboration with overseas partners; and by assessing standards of teaching and learning at subject level. These activities result in reports that are in the public domain.

In order to fulfil its function the QAA will:

- 'work with HEIs to promote and support continuous improvement in the quality and standards of provision;
- provide clear and accurate information to students, employers and others about the quality and standards of higher education provision;
- work with HEIs to develop and manage the qualifications framework;
- advise on the granting of degree awarding powers and university title;
- facilitate the development of benchmark information to guide subject standards;
- promulgate codes of practice and examples of good practice;
- operate programmes of review of performance at institutional and programme level.'

(QAA 1997)

External peers employed and trained by QAA review courses make judgements based on the self-assessment submitted by the university and taking as their frame of reference the student experience. The self-assessment is an evaluation of the quality of the student learning experience, measured against the aims and objectives that the subject provider sets for the education of its students in nursing. The result is a score of 1–4 (1 equating to 'does not meet objectives' to 4 'fully meets') in six areas similar to those described for curriculum validation. The period 1998–2000 was the first time that all nursing programmes had been reviewed in the higher education section (QAA 1997).

Subject benchmarks

All subject areas will have a set of subject benchmarks written before the next round of QAA review. During 2000 the nursing and midwifery subject benchmarks are being formulated by a group of nursing academics, service personnel and professional bodies and are being consulted on before being published.

Subject benchmark information provides a set of principles shared by the subject community. They can then be used as a basis for discourse when quality and standards are reviewed. They should be broad statements, which represent the general expectations about standards for the award in a particular subject area. They should encapsulate the conceptual framework that gives nursing its identity and coherence, and state the intellectual capability and understanding, the techniques and skills associated and the intellectual demand and challenge appropriate to the level of study. This is a challenging task for the nursing group due to the ongoing debate on competencies required for registered practitioners and the different academic levels that are available.

Programme specification

One of the recommendations of the The National Committee of Inquiry into Higher Education, chaired by Lord Dearing (DfEE 1997) was that HEIs make the outcome of the learning more explicit to students and the wider public. The planning team responsible for the course should have articulated a course specification in language that is understandable. This will aid internal and external evaluation of the quality and standards.

National qualification framework

The QAA is developing a national qualification framework, one for Scotland and one for the rest of the UK. This work also follows recommendations from the Dearing Report (DfEE 1997). The framework will rationalise the present situation by developing consistent and coherent structures within which all higher education qualifications and their standards will be located. The aim is to progressively implement the framework from 2001 to 2006. The course will have to adhere to this framework and be judged against it.

The professional and statutory bodies (PSBs)

Nursing, midwifery and health visiting programmes also have to comply with PSB rules and regulations and are subject to quality review from these bodies. The national boards have the responsibility to validate, approve and review institutions and their programmes on behalf of the United Kingdom Central Council for Nursing, Midwifery and Health Visiting (UKCC). This will change in 2001, as the recommendations of the *Report on the Review of the Nurses and Midwives and Health Visiting Act* (DoH 1997b) into the workings of the statutory bodies comes into effect. The advent of parliamentary devolution to Scotland, Wales and Northern Ireland means that the four national boards will change and function differently. Whatever new bodies come into existence they will still be charged with ensuring that the programmes that are approved adhere to statutory requirements and enable graduates to be fit for practice.

The national boards conjointly with the university validate and approve the specialist practitioner degree. It is good practice to involve the institute's designated education officer (DEO) and specialist subject lead officer from the national board in the early development of the new curriculum. Once approved DEOs will monitor on-going quality of the course against the PSB standards (ENB 1997) in the annual monitoring review (AMR). The course will be reviewed at least once in a five-year cycle. The designated education officer will take evidence from the university's own quality assurance documentation, make practice placement visits and meet with mentors, students, employers, users and teachers in order to make judgements. Each year a report against the standards will be produced for the nursing programmes that have been reviewed; these reports over the five-year period give a comprehensive picture of the quality of the institution. If during this process the programme and/or the institution do not meet any of the standards then action will need to be taken and a date set for re-review. The professional statutory bodies have the right to remove approval of a programme. Frequent dialogue, regular visits and communication between the university and the DEO should prevent this happening and should lead to synergy between fitness for award and fitness for practice. On-going changes to the programme will also need to be reported and, if major, agreed to by the DEO. Different officers have various ways of achieving this.

Having a number of external organisations involved in quality assurance of the same provision can put undue pressure on to the university and staff in repetition of the production of evidence and numerous visits. The best way to prevent this is for the organisations to talk to each other and utilise each other's findings. This was evidenced in the joint QAA and ENB visits in 1998–2001, with the Board being members of the QAA review team, reviewers undertaking parts of the AMR process and the QAA using evidence from Board reports on practice.

Commissioners (funders) of education

The NHS commissions education programmes through locally-based workforce development confederations. Membership of the confederation is representative of the employers of health care staff from Trusts, Health Authorities, private and voluntary agencies and social services from the confederation's locality.

The specialist practitioner course will be subject to a contract with the local workforce development confederation. The contract stipulates the number of students, mode of delivery (e.g. part or full time), funding and length of the contract. Most of these contracts contain a quality specification that outlines the quantitative and qualitative data that the confederation requires. It is through these data that the NHSE quality assures the provision they pay for. In the recent paper *A Health Service of all the talents; Developing the NHS workforce* (DoH 2000c), the role of the NHSE in assuring itself of the quality of the programmes and their fitness for purpose is reinforced:

'Delivering this will require close working and constant dialogue at both national and local level so that all parties contribute to the development of genuinely joint working. Such dialogue should help to overcome the concerns expressed to us that training requirements were dominating service provision, and yet that training does not always deliver staff with the skills the NHS require.'

(DoH 2000c, para 5.37)

Again there is a potential for unnecessary repetition in reporting processes. Where there is good practice confederation officers use university documentation, and keep to the minimum that documentation which has to be provided separately. Regular meetings during the year between the contracting parties enable strategic direction and operational issues to be discussed and resolved and confederation officers as members of curriculum planning groups are examples of good joint working.

Employers

Employers are key players in quality assurance because they have a key interest in the knowledge and skills of the staff they employ. They are also active players in the educative process by providing workplace experience and supporting their staff who are mentors. Partnership working between employers, their staff and teachers can be enhanced by activities such as joint planning, development and evaluation of programmes and joint roles in teaching and/or research and practice. It is extremely important that the mentors and teachers work together on planning the curriculum for the specialist practitioner degree, especially in the methods that ensure the reliability and validity of the practice assessment.

Users of service

The input to quality assurance processes from users of the service is growing. Users are now active players in the design of programmes, especially in mental health and maternity care. They are being regularly invited to participate in the teaching and learning of students. An area that is open for future development is user involvement in the assessment of learners and evaluation of the quality of the output. User satisfaction could be an indicator of the success of the educative process.

Quality audit

Auditing their quality assurance systems is another mechanism that HEIs use to ensure the quality of their awards and standards. Many of the external review mechanisms mentioned undertake audit as part of their review by making judgements on whether universities are following their stated quality assurance processes.

Universities also have internal systems of audit based on various methodologies either inbuilt as part of the assurance systems or as a separate activity at either university, faculty, school, division or programme level.

An example of a separate audit is taken from the UNN. A decision was taken to adopt a thematic approach to audit across the university. Four themes were chosen: assessment, learning resources, student support and guidance, and student feedback. The Quality Improvement Academic Standards (QIAS) Committee set up the audits and co-ordinated them through the university's quality and enhancement unit (QEU), with audit teams drawn from across the university. Methodology varied across the audits, with sampling usually from two faculties which had no staff on the audit team. A report of the findings was submitted to QIAS with recommendations for action and was circulated to Faculty Quality Committees (FQCs). Changes to practice were supposed to occur by dissemination to schools/departments. This change was sporadic and only happened effectively when it was seen as part of the audit process and responsibility for and monitoring of action were identified.

Another example based at faculty level was when the Faculty of Health, Social Work and Education (HSWE) at UNN decided to audit all FQC documentation on course development over a five-year period. As a result of this audit and review an IT system was devised that can be used by FQC and course teams to analyse programme evolution, monitor number of changes and ensure that the quality loop on actions from validations and on-going change has been completed

Learning environments should be audited on an annual or bi-annual basis. This includes the placements for students. A model of good practice is evident with the specialist practitioner course at UNN where the environment is audited using a specifically designed audit tool and implemented in partnership with community staff (UNN 1997).

Quality enhancement

Quality enhancement is about constantly endeavouring to improve the quality of courses, standards of teaching and the learning experience for students.

Quality is dependent on the quality of the staff and non-staff resource. Teachers and mentors are key elements in motivating and supporting students. The knowledge and skills of these staff are fundamental to the quality of the learning experience as is the quality of the environment for learning and the library and information systems available to support learning.

Universities should have systems in place to identify the number of staff required and the knowledge and skill they need to perform their role. This is achieved by sound recruitment and selection policies, staff induction and mentoring and annual appraisal that monitors the achievement of objectives and identifies staff development needs. University teachers have time built into their contracts to undertake research and scholarly activity. This is used to undertake research, development of new teaching and learning materials, writing publications and/or clinical activity. Opportunities are afforded for staff to attend internal, national and international conferences in their subject area and to belong to professional/discipline groups.

Mentors undergo initial education into their role, which is enhanced in a variety of ways by regular update sessions, written information and individual visits from teachers.

Identifying and sharing good practice, encouraging innovation in teaching and learning, developing and using evidence-based education, and encouraging staff to reflect and learn from their experience as a teacher/ mentor will all improve the quality of the provision. Many universities have central QEUs whose prime function is to identify quality enhancement strategies and develop, encourage and support on-going improvement within the institution.

A number of universities are introducing peer review and observation in order to enhance teaching and learning. Peer review was introduced in 1998 in the Faculty of Health, Social Work and Education (HSWE) at UNN based on a collaborative and supportive model. A set of guidelines has since been produced on peer review and observation, and these have been translated into an internal university publication (Chalmers 1999). This is an example of how good practice and innovation can be shared across an organisation.

Conclusion

It has only been possible to provide a snapshot of how quality is maintained within higher education institutions. Nevertheless, it is clear that the quality assurance process is an extremely complex area, the success of which is dependent on key stakeholders working together to provide courses of study which prepare practitioners to meet the changing demands of professional practice. During the process of curriculum development, quality and standards have to be developed and implemented in an area subject to continual change and scrutiny. The requirements of the UKCC, ENB, government policy, internal and external quality assurance systems, and local stakeholders must be incorporated into a course which has to be delivered in a limited time span with limited funding, but which must demonstrate innovative approaches to teaching and learning. The current agenda for specialist practitioners is both exciting and challenging; however we must continually strive to work together to develop and deliver innovative courses which ensure that future practitioners are fit for both purpose and practice.

Part 2
Theory and Practice Context

Having dealt in Part 1 with the considerable array of policies that influence mentors and specialist community practitioner students, Part 2 moves on to discussion focused on the theories that relate directly to teaching, the facilitation of learning, student support and the assessment of practice.

The first chapter focuses on learning approaches where theory is integrated with examples from practice. This is followed by reflective practice and naturally (to us) by clinical supervision. The fourth chapter provides an overview of how the ENB Higher Award is applied by one HEI and this Part ends with a weighty chapter concerned entirely with assessing specialist community practitioner students in practice settings.

Chapter 4

Learning Approaches in the Practice Context

Judith Canham and Sue Moore

As this book intends to enable mentors in community settings to develop and enhance their specific role, we made the decision to focus only on those theories and concepts that are relevant to specialist community practitioner students' learning needs. Judith Canham and Sue Moore make sense of the vast array of educational theory by providing a series of case studies taken from real life practice and identifying how practice relates to theory (rather than the other way around). Readers will therefore find that case studies open up the discussions. Although these case studies are about specific disciplines, one role title may easily be substituted for another of your choosing.

Introduction

One of the realities of expert practice is that practitioners are rarely aware of the approaches, theories and concepts that influence and support their practice, integration of theory and practice being automatic (Benner 1984). However, those new to a field need to refer regularly to theory in order to guide practice and to verify the 'rightness' of actions. For those new to mentoring or others needing to update their understanding of educational theory, this chapter offers an integrating approach; specific theory is appraised for its potential value and applicability to specialist practice in the community.

Educational theory is complex and broad ranging and can seem daunting; to counter that, a series of case studies address various aspects of theoretical and conceptual positions in different practice situations. Key concepts and a sample of the main theories are summarised, secondary to the case studies. Although the case studies relate to specific practices, the principles are transferable to most situations. Our intention is that this approach will enable you to make a professional choice about applicability and acceptability, rather than feeling that you ought to adopt this or that theory simply because it is expounded in the literature.

Critical thinking

Without doubt, the greatest benefit of degree level study for the specialist student is the opportunity to develop higher-order thinking skills or 'critical thinking' (Girot 1995) both in theory and practice. With these skills, specialist students can learn to deal with complex practice issues and constant change, drawing on a sound knowledge base to either defend or argue coherently against decisions made in practice. Theoretically, critical thinking skills enable practitioners to promote safe and competent practice through knowledgeable and balanced reviews of all aspects of practice on a continuous basis. The agenda for critical thinking includes all aspects of the practice and the practitioner's role and one of the challenges for mentors is determining for students the minutiae of what practice is and what practitioners do. Unless this is clearly articulated the student may not have any real substance with which to 'generate opinions, see possibilities, discriminate intelligently, be creative and identify new ideas' (Burnard 1990, p. 33). The second challenge is to provide an atmosphere that actively encourages students to question both practice and practitioners and analyse what could or should be done against what is being done.

Promoting and developing critical thinking is not always an easy process as a number of nurses entering specialist practitioner education will have been socialised into nursing practices that actively discouraged critical thought (Melia 1987). Part of the initial learning process in HEI is encouraging concrete thinkers to question actively the primacy of taught material and to develop their own sources of relevant 'information'. As this process initially disturbed lecturers who were used to being the fount of all knowledge, so critical thinkers arriving in practice may upset those practitioners who are content with the ways 'things have always been'. Even though specialist students recognise why preference for the known occurs, they still need to question, to ask for justification and to be creative in order to demonstrate that they can make a difference to health care practices. However difficult the journey might be, a new NHS that demands improvement in the health of the UK populace (DoH 1997a; DoH 1999a), will find it hard to tolerate a lack of critical thought about practice in the very practitioners charged with the delivery of quality care. One of the major responsibilities of mentors is ensuring that critical thinking is actively encouraged, but as the mentor is immersed in practice, promoting critical thinking may mean arguing against one's own accepted wisdom. It is apparent that mentors need to develop critical thinking abilities that at least measure up to those of specialist practitioner students.

The mentor's role

To describe the exact learning needs of specialist practitioner students in nursing and health visiting is impossible as specialist community practitioner roles not only vary from practice to practice but also adapt to patient/client need on a daily basis. Job descriptions will state employers' expectations and the ENB preparation for roles, but it is only mentors who can define the minutiae of what specialist community practitioner students need to learn. By this we mean that although the ENB (1995) states that the specialist practitioner in general practice nursing will 'assess, diagnose and treat specific diseases in accordance with agreed medical/nursing protocols' (ENB 1995, 23.2, p. 25), the interpretation of 'specific disease' and the evaluation of the appropriateness of 'medical/nursing protocols' demand the expertise of an experienced specialist practitioner, the mentor. The wealth of detail provided by the UKCC, ENB and university handbooks cannot begin to substitute for the knowledge of an appropriately qualified mentor.

Similarly, knowing the student, their relevant history, aspirations and preferred learning style(s) in the context of expected learning outcomes is the way in which the mentor can identify the most appropriate approach to adopt for facilitating a student's practice placement. Although this implies that the mentor alone should select a theory for teaching and learning, it will become clear that there are implicit rules; a 'non-adult' approach is inappropriate and behavioural techniques should be used with caution within an overall approach that respects and values the mature student and the needs of specialist practice.

In order to be educationally prepared for their future role, specialist students require the expertise of mentors able to:

- Articulate the complexity of specialist practice
- Enable the appropriate transfer of previously acquired skills, knowledge and attributes
- Teach and facilitate learning to meet the needs of the student and specialist practice
- Assess acquired competencies at the specialist practitioner level.

Although some taught skills and knowledge are universal, teaching and learning skills acquired previously cannot be assumed to be automatically transferable to specialist practice, especially in community settings. Community mentors should be versed in the facilitation of specific learning for mature, responsible students, that satisfies public and organisational need for competent specialist practice.

Competency

Rani is new to health visiting (HV) having previously worked as a midwife. She started in practice in September and by December her mentor (Alan) was concerned that Rani wasn't functioning at an appropriate level. Alan articulated this as, 'Rani is acting as a midwife not a health visitor. She's not completing primary assessments at the appropriate level and has many gaps in her knowledge of developmental assessments.' Alan told Rani of his concerns. Rani was surprised as she felt that her learning in practice was progressing well.

Case study 4.1 Identifying specialist practice competencies

Alan is an experienced health visitor but lacked a learning plan and an approach for facilitating learning and most importantly, failed to think 'student and practice' rather than think purely practice. This distinction is vital. A focus on practice would be appropriate for a qualified practitioner (Jarvis & Gibson 1985); for example, 'does this new health visitor meet the needs of the health visiting service?'. However, that stance cannot be applied to a student health visitor where the question should be, 'do I and practice meet the needs of the student?'. If the current needs of practice assume priority, the needs of the student are likely to be ignored.

Enabling competency

One of Alan's first remedial strategies was to review the course and ENB (1995) outcomes for the student health visitor. He then discussed these and general issues about competency with Rani.

A major part of the mentor role is to *enable* the student to be competent at the specialist practitioner role, which is different from assessing competency. The mentor's facilitation of the development of competencies gives the student the opportunity to learn and to succeed. It is worth noting here that mentors need to ensure that their definition of competency matches that of the HEI. If competency comprises the intent, functions and meaning of a skilled performance (Benner 1984) this would sit well with the specialist student who is required to have a deep understanding of the rationale behind the skilled performance, the range of alternative choices, varying perspectives and approaches.

Competency can also be seen in terms of life-long learning, and the theoretical and practical approaches used to facilitate competency acquirement will determine whether or not learning will be pursued throughout the professional career (Hughes 1994), enjoyable challenges being preferable to mundane task acquisition. In order to facilitate learning of competent practice, the first task is to establish what needs to be learnt. The next step is to determine the period of learning, precise competencies, and priorities for learning, and before going any further, decide on the best method(s) of assessment.

A point for serious consideration is the explication of any hidden agenda that is not written in the course or ENB documents but which is considered professionally essential. This hidden agenda could include such points as 'being flexible', 'using negotiation skills' and 'professional maturity'. If a hidden agenda exists it must be made clear to the student, otherwise learning and assessment become obstacles that the student has no chance of over-coming.

To Alan and Rani the question about defining competencies for health visiting was quickly resolved through ENB and course outcomes; the remaining dilemma was when real competency should occur and how glimmers of competency could be developed. They determined that real competency may only arise in the final weeks of the course but that elements of competency may arise at any time. Alan's role was to ensure that Rani could visualise an arising element and Rani's role was to develop her ability to integrate elements into a coherent whole-competency. The timing and co-ordination of theory and practice learning were important to Rani and Alan as this helped Rani make sense of both aspects simultaneously (Davis 1990; Baillie 1993).

Alan's later analysis of Rani's practice learning provided some useful insights for his own professional development:

'The interesting thing here is that after all my experience I was blaming Rani for her so-called failures, whereas I should have been asking myself what I – the mentor – needed to do. I got a copy of Rani's university timetable and this was really useful as it showed I was expecting far too much. In December they were just moving off family-centred care and other general principles of health visiting. Assessment was the focus for January–February! Because of our little problem I felt there was an urgent need to work on Rani's existing skills and strengths (albeit related to midwifery) and my job was to facilitate their transfer to current practice. We decided jointly that an andragogical approach would be best as she was a highly motivated learner with a wealth of previous learning and experience. As we'd evidently had a communication breakdown, we talked in detail about why this had occurred and ensured that we had the opportunity for an hour's supervision at least once a week. Once we'd started on this proper educational track, issues soon resolved themselves. I learnt a lot from Rani, especially her openness and honesty.'

Rani's view of what had happened was:

'At first I wasn't too sure what Alan wanted from me. I was confused about HV theories but quite happy in practice as I could see that this was what I wanted to do. After Alan said that I wasn't progressing, my confidence plummeted but all credit to him, he apologised and agreed that he'd been expecting too much of me. The next few days were a little uncomfortable but we had a long, forthright talk just before Christmas and decided on a plan of action for January. We also discussed my strengths and really, I knew how to assess in health visiting but at that time I wasn't competent – I didn't think I was! In January both of us knew what I needed to learn in order to develop my competencies. After that it was plain sailing – hard but very interesting. The supervision sessions really helped as every week we talked about my development.'

Adult learning: andragogy

As adults undertaking a new educational programme, specialist students will bring with them a wide range of expertise and knowledge, not only resulting from their formal education but also as a consequence of their personal or professional life experiences. Writers such as Knowles (1990) have attempted to identify the key characteristics of adults as learners, including what appear to be the prime motivators to undertake learning activities. Knowles coined the term andragogy to describe his model of the 'art and science of helping adults to learn' in which he makes the following assumptions:

- Adults are increasingly motivated to be self-directed in their learning, although they can be dependent in some situations. For example, a student may begin their specialist practitioner programme, already expert in medical nursing but lacking the necessary competencies to effectively meet the health needs of clients in community settings. For those who are relative novices in that situation, they are likely to be initially quite dependent on the mentor for guidance and support, although they will increasingly become more self directed as their skills and confidence increase.
- Adults' past experiences are an excellent resource for learning. Therefore, students are likely to learn more effectively if the mentor uses experiential techniques such as critical discourse and problem solving to examine client care planning issues.
- Adults' prime motivation for learning is often related to developing knowledge or skills that will enable them to solve real life problems; for example, to undertake educational activities that enable client-led care.
- Adults' motivation for learning is often related to the ability to apply any new knowledge or skill to their current situation. Therefore, it is vital that the mentor demonstrates the relevance of practice-based learning to the current realities of the practice environment.

Within his discussion of andragogy, Knowles (1990) is describing a student-centred approach to teaching and learning which he contrasts to the traditional pedagogic teaching of children where the teacher would take the lead in deciding what would be learned and how the learning would be undertaken. In the context of specialist practice education, in which a key aim is to facilitate the development of a reflective autonomous practitioner who is capable of self-directed learning, a purely 'teacher'-centred approach would not be appropriate as it would be likely to inhibit rather than promote effective learning. However, McAllister *et al.* (1997) highlight a dilemma inherent in clinical education: that whilst wishing to promote the goals of student autonomy and self-direction, the legal and ethical considerations of client care and the requirement to achieve specific professional competencies dictate that students cannot have complete control over what they should learn, needing the support and guidance of the mentor in working towards increasing autonomy and self-direction in learning activities. A balance may be achieved through student reflection on practice and learning, combined with recognition of professional and public need for specific competencies.

Kim is an experienced mentor/district nurse who was put off by Ruth's requests to 'teach me what I need to know'. Ruth had worked as staff nurse in the community for three years and had completed her Level II studies through a series of modules, paid for by Ruth and undertaken in her own time. Discussion with Ruth identified that in her last practice, the team leader had been 'the boss' with team members being delegated all tasks under the strict supervision of the team leader: 'We'd never dare question her!'

Although during her Level II studies Ruth had been self-determining, she had always felt that others knew best and that she had very little to contribute on an intellectual level.

Ruth was an experienced nurse who demonstrated excellent clinical care and relationships with patients and their carers but she appeared to be limp and malleable in the face of presumed authority. This was also exhibited in her working relationships with general practitioners and other members of the Primary Care Team. She was probably the archetypal good, obedient nurse (Melia 1987; Alavi & Cattoni 1995) but subservience in modern practice was the last thing that Kim wanted to see. Considering the short length of the course, Ruth would have to move quickly from being passive to leading practice, and the mentor-student relationship was the ideal environment to start practising assertiveness, self-determination and pro-activity.

Kim discussed her concerns with Ruth and placed the onus on Ruth to decide what should be done to move her practice forward. Ruth was aware of the skills she needed and knew why she didn't use them; interestingly she put a lot down to laziness – 'there was always someone else to deal with the hassles' – and much to fear of being disliked. Ruth's action plan, agreed by Kim, was that the teaching/learning approach would be humanistic (Rogers 1969) with Ruth being self-directing and Kim facilitative. Within that approach Ruth's first objective was to undertake a self-assessment of all her existing professional skills, knowledge and attributes. There were to be as many strengths as limitations and each point needed to be justified in relation to 'how do I know this?' and planned in relation to 'what do I need to learn and how?'. The second objective was to observe accepted leaders in practice and to note *their* strengths and limitations and particularly if they were disliked or respected. These objectives took precedence over patient care as Ruth had already established her clinical competencies. Ruth set a date for evaluating this part of her learning through discussion with Kim.

The third and most important (and most daunting) objective set by Ruth, was that within four weeks she was going to determine her own small case-load, and select and ask one staff nurse to join her 'team'. Ruth was to delegate to this staff nurse and to Kim.

Case study 4.2 Enabling the development of leadership

The strategy for learning in case study 4.2 mirrors Rogers' (1969) principles of learning; most importantly the atmosphere was safe, even though the objectives were intensely challenging. At the beginning there was little in the way of teaching but a huge learning curve for Ruth. The learning process was monitored by Kim who maintained daily contact and provided clinical supervision on a weekly basis and when required by Ruth (see Chapter 6 for more detail of clinical supervision).

Kim summed up the practice placement as:

> 'Interesting! Ruth still isn't the best leader I've known but she's as good as many and better than some. She's quietly assertive and that makes a nice change here. Adopting a purely humanistic approach may seem to have been a little hard on Ruth but we had no choice given her initial behaviours and the goals she had to achieve. Had we used another approach, say adult learning, we could have achieved her learning objectives but she needed to feel in control, to make choices while at the same time knowing that she was in a really supportive professional relationship. She knew what she had to achieve but that I was there and on her side. The hardest part for me was taking a back seat and letting her make some mistakes. I knew she wouldn't make them with patients, but she did make them. A social worker said, 'Who the hell's that arrogant b. . .?'. I had to feed back to Ruth and she agreed that she'd gone over the top, but she'd been right. It's all a matter of communication at the end of the day and the more you do it the easier it gets. Specialist practice takes experience.'

Ruth's evaluation of her practice was:

> 'A nightmare at first and then just exhausting as I really had to work hard. My worst and best day was when, without prompting, I asked a G grade on another team to stop making comments about a colleague as I found her attitude offensive. I'm not sure who was the most surprised! I've learnt a lot through this type of learning. Although I led my transition, I always knew that Kim was there and supported me. Our supervision sessions were sometimes a bit painful for me but once I'd got the knack, I knew that the issues weren't personal but about the development of this person who could stand up to anyone and say, 'Well OK, yea, I've not done too well but I will do better' or, 'Hey, this is a real person you're talking about, you can't fob them off with this or that, this is the best care . . .'

The humanistic approach

In recent years, the humanistic approach to adult education has been prominent in highlighting the importance of giving the student more control over their learning, and of the teacher/mentor taking a more facilitative approach. It is argued that human beings have a natural potential for growth and development and the role of the teacher/mentor is to facilitate this natural growth. The key to unlocking this natural potential is to give students the necessary control to be more self-directing, so that they develop the transferable skills of learning how to learn, increasingly without the need for close direction by the teacher/mentor.

An influential writer in this humanistic field has been Carl Rogers, who from his background in client-centred psychotherapy went on to develop a student-centred approach to learning. Within the key work *Freedom to Learn* (Rogers 1969) he proposes a number of principles of learning:

- Human beings have a natural potential for learning
- Effective learning takes place when the subject is perceived to be relevant to the student's own life
- Learning is most effective when it takes place in a trusting and non-threatening environment
- Experience is important in promoting effective learning
- Where teacher and student are able to agree aims and clarify roles and responsibilities, this helps to give the student responsible freedom to learn
- Where self evaluation is encouraged, this helps to facilitate student independence, creativity and self reliance.

According to Rogers, the main role of the teacher/mentor is to act as a facilitator of learning, who as well as being a provider of resources for the students should be able to share his feelings with the students. Therefore, the necessary prerequisites of an effective facilitator of learning in the humanistic tradition would be:

- Self-awareness
- Genuineness
- Understanding and empathy
- Acceptance and trust of the students' feelings and views.

Rogers highlights that the learning environment should be nurturing rather than controlling, placing great emphasis on the emotional aspects of learning, which may be helpful in the development of interpersonal skills, reflection and self-awareness in health care education. Also, if mentors are able to foster creativity and independence, then students may be able to be more innovative within their practice settings, in meeting the demands of a dynamic and changing health care environment.

Ceri is a general practice nurse student. She had some experience in practice nursing before commencing the course on a part-time basis. She had recently completed a DipHE Nursing Studies on an independent, part-time basis. She has two young children and is a school governor. Maria is a very experienced general practice nurse and has just completed a short, Level III course for mentors.

In the first week of Ceri's placement, Maria determined that the overall educational approach should be based on andragogy; Ceri was an adult with recent higher education learning experiences. The overall approach should also include cognitivism; as a specialist community practitioner (SCP) student Ceri needed to learn from and through experience. Maria also felt that the humanistic approach had a lot of appeal as the student-mentor relationship was extremely important and Maria wanted to move away from a more traditional, directive approach to teaching and learning.

Maria was concerned about getting her approach muddled but when she discussed her concerns with the university teacher she felt that she could treat educational theories as she treated nursing theories; rarely did one nursing theory meet a client's needs and Maria often used a mix (an eclectic approach). Using this eclectic approach, Maria and Ceri jointly decided on a broad teaching and learning strategy for the entire placement. They then determined that particular learning needs would need particular approaches. For example, when Ceri needed to learn skills, e.g. the management of cervical cytology, there would be the need to adopt some behavioural techniques plus cognitive theory. However overall, andragogical and humanistic theories would dominate the learning process.

As Maria had recently completed mentor preparation, she continued to feel dominated by educational theory until she felt comfortable that she was facilitating Ceri's professional development in an appropriate way. She felt that the theories gave her support and allowed her to plan the different aspects of Ceri's learning needs in specific ways. For example, when Ceri needed to learn a new skill, Maria utilised behaviourist techniques which quickly moved through a series of skill acquisition objectives (Hinchliff 1992) in order to ensure that Ceri's practice was safe. However, as Ceri was studying specialist practice this in itself was not sufficient. Although Maria could have moved through a taxonomy to develop deeper learning (Gagne 1970) she opted to apply a cognitive approach at the same time so that while Ceri was learning new practical skills, she would also be transferring knowledge from the past to the present.

At the end of the placement, Ceri felt that she had received an 'excellent and intensive practice education'. Maria was a little more critical:

> 'At the end of the day, I feel that Ceri did learn from me but the whole time I was overwhelmed by just how much she had to learn and my responsibility to ensure that she was a safe and thinking practitioner at the specialist level. Although I felt bogged down by theory and did frequently get confused, I feel that my use of theories, double-checking and doing lots more reading, helped me and Ceri to know what we were doing. If, say, I hadn't used any particular theory but my own common sense, I may have missed some of the detail that I applied when using a behaviourist technique. It

was little things like listing the complexity of the cervical screening process and ensuring we addressed everything. Just saying, "Well I'm an experienced practice nurse and so I can teach it, using my normal practitioner skills," doesn't make sense to me as my mentor and practitioner skills are different. I'm a good practitioner but I've got a lot to learn about mentorship.

One of the things I've learnt through this is the importance of using an adult approach or perhaps a humanistic approach with all mature students, even if you're using behaviourist techniques. There's no way that I could have asked Ceri to list the responsibilities of the practice nurse in the screening process but I did ensure that she knew them through our discussion sessions; I knew the list! It was incredibly important to reflect on our progress on a weekly basis so that the whole thing was a joint endeavour and not just a teaching exercise. Now I feel that I can start to ignore the theory tags and concentrate more on my next student's learning needs, the most appropriate way to facilitate learning, methods and styles, and then check what I was planning in relation to theory.'

Case study 4.3 Utilising educational approaches to facilitate learning

The behavioural approach

In contrast to the andragogical perspective, which emphasises the role of conscious internal motivating forces in learning, behaviourists stress the importance of stimuli in the external environment in shaping behaviour; learning is defined as a response to a stimulus, which results in a relatively permanent change in observable behaviour. The emphasis is on the product of the learning activity (i.e. a change in behaviour), rather than on the whole learning process.

One of the most influential writers who proposed a behavioural explanation of learning was Gagne (1970), who identified a hierarchy of learning of eight stages, moving from a simple stimulus response to complex problem solving. These stages are signal learning, stimulus-response, chaining, verbal association, discrimination learning, concept learning, rule learning and problem solving. The structuring of the learning experience, particularly at the lower levels of the hierarchy, is very much under the control of the teacher/mentor, with the role of the student being a fairly passive one with limited opportunities for self-direction. In the case of specialist students it is clear that behavioural techniques alone will not be able to provide the student with the wide range of skills, knowledge and attributes that make up competency at the specialist practitioner level. However, some students may need to learn specific psychomotor skills related to the management of clinical care, and in these situations Gagne's (1970) approach may still be useful albeit within an overall approach that respects adult learning.

The cognitive approach

Cognitive psychologists argue that it is the internal cognitive processing of information that is important in bringing about learning (Messick 1976). The Gestalt school of cognitive psychology proposes that people tend to perceive information as a whole, rather than in isolated bits in order to try and make sense of it. Taking this view, a student's perception of a learning activity undergoes some cognitive restructuring, so that the elements of the activity are perceived in a new relationship and a solution is achieved by insight when the elements are perceived to come together. A more complex explanation of cognitive learning has been described by Ausubel (1968) who argues that learning takes place as a result of an interaction between new information and existing ways of processing information as a cognitive activity (cognitive structuring). For example, learning is brought about through an interaction of new information and existing cognitive structures that results in the formation of more detailed structures. For Ausubel, meaningful learning (as opposed to learning by rote) is not a passive process as the student has to engage actively in the learning activity for effective learning to occur.

Using Ausubel's approach in health care education, the curriculum needs to be structured so that new learning builds on logically from what has gone before, moving from more foundational concepts and principles to more complex material, so that learning increases in progressive stages. The role of the mentor in using this approach would be initially to help the student appreciate the foundational concepts and principles of specialist practice, for example the management of client care in a community setting. These could be applied by students meeting the specific health needs of their client group in practice and could be evaluated with the mentor, so that new insights and meaningful learning could be achieved through the experience of applying these principles in practice and cognitively reflecting on them.

The learning environment: organising opportunities for learning

---

Jane is an occupational health nurse (OHN) and a new mentor. 'To be honest I wasn't too sure about having a student for a whole year partly because I thought I'd be shattered and secondly because I didn't think the NHS was a totally suitable learning experience as it lacks the industrial and broad knowledge base the OHN needs. However, once I placed myself in a facilitating role rather than the more traditional teaching role I'd been used to, I found that I could enable Ian to learn all that he needed to. We were lucky enough to meet before the course started as the Occupational Health Department (OHD) is very keen on quality. We brainstormed what skills, knowledge and attributes were required of any OHN, matched these with the university aims and ended up with three lists:

- Ian's existing skills, knowledge and attributes
- Knowledge, attributes and skills that could be met here
- Skills that would have to be learned elsewhere.

The skills that I couldn't address were in fact quite few and were mainly around occupational injuries and hazards encountered in industry, and working with groups of workers outside the NHS. As I belong to an OHN support group I was able to negotiate with colleagues in industry to support Ian for two two-week planned periods of learning.

Case study 4.4 Using learning opportunities

In case study 4.4 it is obvious that although some skills had to be met elsewhere, knowledge could be acquired through Jane's appropriate facilitation of the entire learning process. Knowledge of the strengths and limitations of the narrow learning environment and an appreciation of wider resources for learning can be vital to the student's proper development. Surprisingly the importance of the breadth of the learning environment is understated in most texts for nurse education but this may relate to the focus of these texts (pre-registration) where the 'normal' environment is considered to be the 'controlled' ward. The community rarely has such natural barriers and the learning environment includes the client population, the building(s), professional and lay staff, external resources that can be utilised and where the student learns (i.e. in the patient's home). A community, practice, school or workplace profile is one way of identifying learning opportunities within practice, and the mentor has a responsibility to ensure that an up-to-date profile of learning opportunities is available (ENB 1997). However, day-to-day practice situations can also produce a myriad of learning opportunities that cannot be detailed such as:

> 'An impromptu discussion relating to client choice and employment regulations following a student nurse's reluctance to let the OHN take blood.'

An additional factor influencing the learning environment is that mentors cannot wholly forgo their practice commitments, because of professional responsibility and because students are there to learn within and from that practice. Although education may be described as a 'planned series of incidents' (Jarvis 1983), teaching in the community also takes place on an opportunistic basis and may take place in some rather unusual places; planning an appropriate learning environment for students requires flexibility and in some cases, as Jane discovered, ingenuity:

Tuesday 9th: Disaster – staff off sick – everyone very harassed and tetchy – work awful – meningitis jabs have to be completed today!

- It may be a good experience for the student to be a part of the chaos and learn from it – how staff act – how to prioritise. Problem is that no one will

45

have any time for the student. Depending on the student's level of experience they may be more of a hindrance than a help.
- It could be appropriate to suggest to the student that s/he uses the day to spend time with another agency or service. This might be difficult to arrange at such short notice and will increase my stress levels. If the student has something that s/he could organise that may be better.
- Provide personal study time. Sounds a bit of a cop out. Has the student got some specific pressing study?
- Is there some task or project that has been put off for a while? Is the student capable of doing this?
- Give some specific directed study. For instance evaluate the uptake of immunisation and vaccination for the last student nurse cohort.

I am not going to suggest that any one of the five options in case study 4.4 is best, but I hope that they demonstrate that even a disaster can be turned into a learning opportunity. Whatever is decided, the student needs to be in full agreement and there is an absolute need to spend time at a later date reflecting on the experience and determining how valuable it was.

Ian was at first a little disappointed to be placed in the NHS as his career plan was to work in a large industry. However, by the end of the course he felt that he had learnt the principles of OHN and was sufficiently competent to be successful in his application to work in industry as a member of an OHN team:

'I hope that soon I'll be able to take a lead role but realise that although I'm safe and competent I still have a lot to learn. Working in the NHS was interesting and I was surprised that the business ethic isn't just restricted to industry. The planned placements were very useful but I had to put a lot in. After the two weeks I had to evaluate the benefits of the placement and discuss with Jane what I'd learnt so I had to be really focused when I was there.
    All in all I feel that I was able to use some of the skills I'd learnt in A&E and rescued some older skills from general nursing. This meant that although the situation was brand new I felt I had something to contribute. In the NHS we had a spillage, with some minor eye irritations, and Jane asked me for advice on evidence-based practice. She could have been testing me but I think it was a genuine request for my expertise.'

Jane remains a little cautious about being a mentor as she feels some pressure from the commitments of her professional role:

'Everyone in the team pulls together and when Ian was on placement, they tried to take some work off me, but this isn't a perfect world and at times things went pear-shaped. Ian was new to OHN which meant that he needed constant support for the first few months but one of my colleagues pointed out that at times he could support Ian's learning with me keeping overall responsibility. I checked this out with the university and we decided that if I judged my colleague to be an appropriate support mentor, why not? I also used my professional judgement about the other placements as I had to decide if they were good enough for Ian. I used the practice audit for that and then wrote a list of objectives for Ian to learn in those placements. The OHN support group proved to be very useful not just for the placements but also for providing some vital support for me!

Having a workplace profile and a broader resource profile was really good. I knew that we didn't have all the resources to meet Ian's needs, but it identified gaps and potential problems for teaching and learning a complete OHN service. The other thing that happened was that this close examination of professional practice acted as a form of informal audit – allowed me the opportunity to update the profile! Overall I think having a student keeps you up to date.

I'll probably have a student again next year but will also encourage my colleagues to be mentors.'

Students' learning styles

The case studies suggest that each of the educational theories/learning approaches would seem to have something to offer the mentor as potential strategies that could be used to promote more effective student learning within practice. However, experience has shown that even when using what would seem to be the most appropriate approach, some students would appear not to learn as effectively as others. Research undertaken by Marton and Saljo (1984) demonstrates that it is the student's internal or external motivation that affects their style of learning, resulting in either a deep or surface approach to learning. Students who use a deep approach are those who are internally motivated to find personal meaning and understanding through their learning activities; for example, students wanting to develop knowledge and skills in order to improve their practice. Students who use a surface approach to learning are those who were externally motivated to memorise just enough information to pass the assessment or gain the qualification. Effective learning that has a lasting impact is likely to result from using a deeper approach rather than a superficial one, and fortunately most specialist students have immense internal motivation.

Relational theory

Recently, research has suggested that effective learning depends on the relationship between the student, the learning environment, the learning task, teaching methods, assessments, and vitally the student's perceptions of and pre-conceptions about these (Cust 1996). This is likely to affect whether the student will adopt a deep or surface approach to a particular learning situation. For example, students who experience courses which require large amounts of factual information to be recalled for assessment purposes, are likely to adopt a surface approach to learning which will involve memorising key facts to be represented within the assessment. This may be true even for students who would normally have a deeper approach to learning, as it is the way in which the course and assessment methods are structured that influences the student's perceptions of what is valued, and consequently what they believe the learning task requires of them (Entwistle & Ramsden 1983).

In contrast, professional education courses that emphasise the importance of reflection, in order to enhance both client care and promote continuous professional development, are much more likely to encourage a deeper approach to learning, especially if the assessment of practice also formally rewards this. However, some students need help to develop a deeper approach to learning if their previous learning style has been more superficial. It has been suggested that a problem-based approach to teaching can facilitate a deeper approach to learning (Cust 1996), if the teacher can help students to appreciate the relevance of the subjects covered and provide sufficient structure and guidance for them confidently to seek possible solutions. It would appear that mentors are ideally placed to use a problem-based approach with their students in order to facilitate a deeper approach to learning. They have an up-to-date knowledge of real-life client problems and practice issues that could be used to pose relevant problems for students to investigate. This would help students to integrate and test theory in practice and develop appropriate competencies related to their areas of specialist practice, through the investigation of real-life client problems and possible courses of action.

Theory-practice integration

The need for theory-practice integration is vital in the provision of quality care and rather than these being viewed as separate entities they should be considered as one element with different perspectives. To say a theory must be applied in practice is inappropriate; to ask what is the best theory for practice is more helpful. Students may observe specific practices before that specific theory is addressed in any detail, especially as one of the unique aspects of community nursing practice is that any patient/client could present at any time (Andrews 1991). One could easily ask either 'how are theories of palliative care applied in practice?' or 'what has theory got to say about applied palliative care?'. In the first case, the student would 'have' the theories and then question practice; in the second case the student would 'have' the practice and then question theory. However, in this second case mentors should be aware that they may need to be the theory source as they are eminently more flexible in what they can 'teach' than university colleagues restricted by time-tables and rooms.

The application of educational theory

One of the most important issues coming through most of the case studies is the need for students to work towards a mature, responsible stance, best achieved through a student-focused, adult-centred approach. The use of experiential learning (Cernick & Evans 1992), problem solving and problem-based learning (Cust 1996) are all strategies appropriate to learning in and through professional practice. The student will be respected and feel valued and will be able to apply those concepts to the nurse-patient relationship.

Schön (1987) talks about the 'ego trip' of teachers who just want to teach and we can be in no doubt that teaching adults is about facilitating learning; the application of a pedagogical approach is never a feasible approach for specialist students. Traditional methods of education (pedagogic approaches; didactic transmission) may perpetuate inequalities in society – gender, race and age (Hughes 1994) – and as nurse education is within traditional seats of learning (HEI), mentors need to be cautious about the value placed on HEI methods. In HEI, students may be restricted in their ability to take an active part in the learning process (for example in lectures) and may not develop a good teacher-student relationship; this constraint to adult learning disappears in practice where the student can be fully active in the learning process (Cernick & Evans 1992).

Summary

The gulf between the old and new approaches to teaching and learning for specialist practice is vast. The mentor is no longer the fount of all knowledge but a resource that needs to be tapped appropriately. Preferred approaches (humanistic, andragogical, cognitive) use the student and the student's practice to the full though none are an easy option. The student has the responsibility for learning supported by a knowledgeable and approachable mentor who ensures that knowledge, skills and attributes can be learnt through finding a way that suits both the student and the course outcomes. Within this seemingly free approach to learning there is considerable structure, imposed as specialist students have a limited time to achieve set outcomes. Structure applied utilising mentors' understanding of the entire teaching and learning process should enable students to 'see' what they have learnt and understand how long or short the rest of the journey will be.

Chapter 5
Reflective Practice

Joanne Bennett

There can be no doubt that the ability to reflect and apply reflection in practice is an expectation of the specialist community practitioner and of students undertaking professional awards. However, reflection is not an easy skill and art to learn; mentors may struggle as much as students, yet will be expected to guide reflection in and on practice. To assist the learning process, this chapter provides an overview of reflection before progressing to 'critical incident analysis' that can be applied in both the HEI and in practice.

Introduction

The concept of reflection has become a common topic of discussion within nursing, particularly in the climate of clinical effectiveness; it is a term that is often easier to conceptualise than to convert into everyday practice. There are numerous reasons for this, which include having the legitimised time and space in the working day to enable the practitioner to reflect in a purposeful way, and to do so in a supportive environment with colleagues who value the process. Perhaps of more importance is having the opportunity to develop skills in reflection, as reflection 'in' and 'on' practice is not easy (Schön 1987). It can be an extremely uncomfortable, painful and stressful process, particularly when traditional practice is being challenged.

Work with both pre-registration and post-registration students at undergraduate and post-graduate level has reinforced the notion that reflection is a learned process, one that requires guidance, time and support from experienced teachers, mentors and/or colleagues. It is insufficient to simply provide the students with literature on the subject without assisting them to develop strategies and techniques to put this into practice. The importance of this was highlighted through personal experience. As a nurse teacher in the late 1980s, I was fortunate to be provided with the opportunity to work alongside two experienced colleagues who guided and supervised me through the process of using reflective strategies as part of my own learning and development as well as with student nurses. Development of skills and confidence in the use of reflection is arguably crucial to all staff engaging in the process, whether this is from a personal perspective or with students, colleagues or service users.

The purpose of this chapter is to offer some insights into how to use a

50

reflective approach with specialist practitioner students. It is not my intention to enter into lengthy debate about the concept of reflection, as there are numerous texts available which have accomplished this. Nor will I assume that all readers have a grasp of the concept. I will therefore begin by introducing some basic ideas that are intended to stimulate thought. Some of the techniques that have been used to encourage reflection with specialist practitioner students will then be discussed. The critical incident provided by a student district nurse will be central to this. Consideration will then be given to the value, or otherwise, of these approaches. It is important to point out that I am not advocating that reflection has all of the answers to the problems faced by practitioners. It is simply one strategy, which can be used for a number of purposes. Evaluation studies on the benefits of this process are scarce and further evidence does need to be produced to determine the real value of this process.

Reflection

For those readers who are relatively new to the concept of reflection, one of the most widely quoted definitions is that of Boyd and Fales (1983), who suggest that:

> 'Reflection is the process of internally examining and exploring an issue of concern, triggered by an experience, which creates and clarifies meaning in terms of self, and which results in a changed perspective.'

This definition has similarities to that of Boud *et al.* (1985) who state that reflection is:

> 'A complex and deliberate process of thinking about and interpreting experience in order to learn from it.'

It may be worth noting that not all learning arises from issues of concern in practice. It is equally important to explore positive experiences and encourage practitioners to begin to articulate what constitutes 'best practice' and to share this with others. It should also be recognised that some of the techniques that are used to facilitate reflection involve examining and learning from the experiences of others as well as one's own. However, the way in which we reflect and make sense of an experience is very much dependent on our views of knowledge and knowledge generation.

This in itself is a complex area and Taylor (1998) suggests that in relation to nursing it may be helpful to think about three broad, yet arbitrary, categories of knowledge that can be described as empirical, interpretive and critical. He describes empirical knowledge as that which is generated and tested through the use of the scientific method, whilst describing the common features of interpretive and critical knowledge as being context dependent and subjective in nature. He goes on to argue that the main differences lie in the intentions of knowledge generation. Whilst all three categories can bring about change, the way in which this occurs is different. For example, empirical knowledge can supposedly shift and change human thoughts about facts; interpretive knowledge may help raise people's awareness and provide new insights which could lead to actions to accommodate these new insights; and the intention of critical knowledge is to bring about change through getting people to work together to solve problems. Understanding of this complex area and its relationship to reflection may be enhanced if we briefly review the nature of knowledge from an historical perspective and how this relates to nursing.

Historical perspective

Until quite recently, those involved in the education of nurses in both the academic and practice setting traditionally tended to favour knowledge derived from a scientific academic base (empirical knowledge). This knowledge was simply transmitted by the teacher to the student who was then left to put it into practice. It was this form of scientific knowledge that Schön (1987) spoke of when he used the term 'technical rationality'. Technical rationality has its roots in positivism and the scientific method of enquiry. In its extreme form, the concern was about that which was observable, testable and objective. Alongside the importance placed on the scientific method grew the opinion that science could be used to solve human problems. Professionals came to be seen as the vehicle to apply principles of a science to practical situations. The profession of medicine became the prototype for this approach, and eventually other groups, such as nursing, began to copy. This was partly as a result of nursing striving to obtain the status and characteristics of a profession.

However, Schön (1987) describes how from 1963 onwards both the general public and the professionals were becoming increasingly aware of the limitations of the professions. One of the reasons for this was that despite adopting a scientific approach, professionals were failing to solve the many problems evident in society. At this time there was a growing awareness of the uncertainty, complexity and instability of practice situations which did not fit neatly into a model of technical rationality. For example, under the technical rationality model problems are solved through the application of rules and principles derived from a scientific base to practice. This however assumes that problems present themselves in neat little boxes and are unrelated to time and context. As the example in case study 5.1 illustrates, practice is complex, ambiguous and messy and rarely, if ever, fits into a neat box.

As Schön (1987) identifies, the technical rationality model ignores the problem setting stage and the complexity of this, and depends on agreement about the end to the problem. He goes on to argue that technical rationality alone is insufficient to explain the complexity of professional practice. As well as the skills which professionals clearly acquire from practice, Schön suggests that professionals are knowledgeable in a different way. He talks about how we cannot always say what we know as our knowing is tacit/implicit in our patterns of action. He suggests that in our day-to-day behaviour we reveal a kind of knowing that does not stem from books or theories; it is a knowing in action which has the following properties:

- Actions, recognitions and judgements which we know how to carry out spontaneously; we do not have to think about them
- We are often unaware of having learned to do these things; we simply find ourselves doing them
- We are usually unable to describe the knowing which our actions reveal.

This is clearly a complex area. On the one hand we have a form of knowledge developed in research centres at universities, which often bears no relationship to the reality of professional practice. On the other we have knowledge derived from experience which is context specific yet we are often at a loss when trying to explain it. There are a range of reflective strategies which encourage practitioners to select from the theories they have learned that which is most appropriate to the situation they face. In doing so, this knowledge will be developed by practitioners to solve individual problems, thus contributing to their personal store of experience. As well as this, the strategies used encourage practitioners to describe, share and develop their personal knowledge so that it becomes more widely available to other practitioners. Through this sharing, practitioners are provided with new insights which lead to both personal and collective change.

Reflective frameworks

There are many frameworks to draw on, all having both strengths and limitations (e.g. Carper 1978; Meizerow 1981; Gibbs 1988; Atkins & Murphy 1993). Although there are numerous reflective frameworks available of differing levels of complexity, Atkins and Murphy (1993) suggest that it is possible to identify three key stages in the process:

(1) An awareness of uncomfortable feelings and thoughts
(2) Critical analysis – to include the examination of feelings and knowledge
(3) The development of new perspectives.

This is perhaps the case with many reflective frameworks; however there are now some that acknowledge that not all experiences/incidents are negative, e.g. Smith & Russell (1991, 1993). This model utilises critical incidents to help practitioners develop their ability to evaluate critically the strengths and limitations of theoretical frameworks to practice situations, as well as beginning to encourage practitioners to articulate knowledge embedded in practice. When used in the classroom, incidents are selected which are significant for group learning. However, the process can be used on an individual basis through the use of a diary and/or in the practice setting with the mentor and/or academic teacher.

What is critical incident analysis?

Critical incident analysis was a technique first used by Flanagan in 1954 to gather information about both effective and ineffective behaviour of airline pilots on designated flying missions. Pilots were asked to report their observations about their own and other people's behaviour through critical incidents. These were then analysed in relation to the ways in which decisions and choices were made. Using this method Flanagan was able to uncover important aspects of the job performance, identifying stressors and conditions that either impaired or improved performance. From this information he was able to develop criteria for effective leadership as well as specific training needs (Smith & Russell 1993). He also used the technique to categorise student nurse's performance. Benner (1984) adapted the technique to explore the shift from novice to the expert nurse.

The benefits of using this technique with both pre- and post-registration nursing students are numerous, and include:

- The development of skills in reflection
- The facilitation of the integration of theory and practice
- The encouragement of the student to evaluate both the strengths and limitations of theoretical frameworks
- Helping to uncover knowledge embedded in practice
- Helping the student to identify opportunities for practice development
- A means of developing evidence-based practice
- Helping the student to learn how to make decisions under uncertain conditions (Smith & Russell 1991).

Analysis of critical incidents therefore provides students with the opportunity to reflect with other professional colleagues (mentor, peer group, teachers) on particular or similar incidents and explore personal, group and/or theoretical viewpoints which might be helpful in enhancing understanding, as well as providing useful strategies for dealing with similar incidents in the future (see Fig. 5.1 for guidelines).

Guidelines for recording a critical incident

Students are encouraged to write as if they were making a diary entry or writing to a close friend. Issues of confidentiality are addressed and ground rules are set when working in a group. The accounts are anonymous, although students may choose to own them. Many students use this method of recording with personal learning diaries. They may then choose to share the diary entry with the mentor or university teacher in a clinical supervision session, or with their peer group during a structured session on critical incident analysis.

When working with the group, the incidents are collected one week in advance of the session to enable academic staff to undertake a preliminary analysis of emergent themes.

Students are issued with the following guidelines:

A critical incident is any incident that made an emotional impact. It may be in your interactions with a patient, relative or colleague. It could be an incident which:

- Went unusually well
- Was particularly demanding
- You found difficult to handle
- You feel your or another member of staff's intervention made a significant difference to the outcome of care.

What to include in the description:

- The context in which the incident occurred
- Details of what happened
- Thoughts about your concerns at the time. What did you think about? What did you feel about what was happening?
- What you found most demanding about the incident
- Why the incident is important to reflect on.

Fig. 5.1 Guidelines for recording a critical incident.

A single incident may be selected if it is particularly significant to the group. Regardless of whether the incidents are used in a group or on an individual basis, the process of analysis is the same.

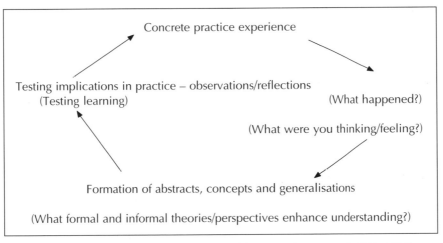

Fig. 5.2 Experiential learning cycle (adapted from Smith & Russell 1991, 1993).

The process is aided through the analysis of responses to various questions:

- What happened in the incident?
- How can it be explained?
- What other formal and informal theories and perspectives are there which help to shed light on the experience/incident?
- What have I learned from this reflection?

These questions are used as triggers at various stages of a reflective cycle (see Fig. 5.2).

Although this model is simple and easy to use, when initially engaging with this process it is often helpful to have more detailed cues such as those provided in Johns' model of structured reflection (Johns 1995). This model consists of a series of questions which help the practitioner to focus on the experience in a meaningful way (see Fig. 5.3).

Regardless of which reflective framework is selected, the starting point is always an account of the experience or critical incident.

Core question – What information do I need in order to learn through this experience?
Cue questions:

1.0   Description of experience
    1.1   Phenomenon – Describe the 'here and now' experience
    1.2   Causal – What essential factors contributed to this experience?
    1.3   Context – What are the significant background factors to this experience?
    1.4   Clarifying – What is the key process (for reflection) in this experience?
2.0   Reflection
    2.1   What was I trying to achieve?
    2.2   Why did I intervene as I did?
    2.3   What were the consequences of my actions for:
        ● myself?
        ● the patient/family?
        ● the people I work with?
    2.4   How did I feel about the experience when it was happening?
    2.5   How did the patient feel about it?
    2.6   How do I know how the patient felt about it?
3.0   Influencing factors
    3.1   What internal factors influenced my decision-making?
    3.2   What external factors influenced my decision-making?
    3.3   What sources of knowledge did/should have influenced my decision-making?
4.0   Could I have dealt better with the situation?
    4.1   What other choices did I have?
    4.2   What would be the consequences of those choices?
5.0   Learning
    5.1   How do I now feel about this experience?
    5.2   How have I made sense of this experience in the light of past experiences and future practice?
    5.3   How has this experience changed my ways of knowing:
        ● empirical?
        ● aesthetic?
        ● ethical?
        ● personal?

Fig. 5.3   Model of structured reflection (Carper 1978; Johns 1995).

Analysis of critical incident

Professional practice is characterised by complexity, ambiguity and uncertainty, with specialist practitioners facing competing and conflicting pressures on an almost daily basis. The problems and challenges faced by the specialist practitioner rarely fit into neat boxes or have simple solutions. This uncertainty is aptly demonstrated in the following account provided by a district nursing student.

'The following incident took place on a routine visit with my mentor. The patient in question had been diagnosed with an inoperable tumour in her bronchus, and she was now in a terminal condition. She was a very depressed lady who had mentally lost the will to live and required a great deal of mental stimulation to perform the very minimum of tasks. Her elderly husband, with the help of social services home care visits twice daily, cared for her.

The day in question was a Monday. On arrival at the house the husband appeared very ill and stated that he was 'off his legs' and had been all weekend. Routine investigations were carried out and it was found that his blood pressure was very low, his appetite had subsided and he felt very sleepy. His wife was unable to perform the minimum of tasks and home care had taken it upon them to increase the visits to four times a day. Assistance was given by my mentor and myself to make both the husband and the wife comfortable.

The GP was informed and a visit requested. I informed the patients that I would return later that day to find out what had happened. I returned after lunch to find the situation deteriorating. Both the husband and wife required further assistance, and I felt that unless some extra input was given the situation would reach crisis point. The GP visited and prescribed antibiotics for a urinary tract infection, without either testing the urine or requesting a sample to be sent to the lab. I felt very let down by the GP. I did not think that he had got to the root of the problem; I was not happy with his decision.

When I returned to the clinic I discussed events with my mentor and asked her advice and opinion whether extra help should be implemented via social services and the health trust under the umbrella of a continual care package. She agreed that it would be a very good idea, as these systems cover patients with a terminal illness for a period of fourteen weeks prior to review. It seemed the obvious choice, as it was clear that this lady was not going to live that long.

I contacted the GP and asked his permission; he refused to sanction the extra care saying that the lady would still be here at Christmas. We were allowed, as nurses, to increase social services care for a couple of days, until the husband recovered. I remember feeling very angry with the GP. How could anybody say that a terminally ill lady would still be here at Christmas? The nursing team felt very anxious that the situation would reach crisis point.

Throughout the week the situation did deteriorate. The lady agreed to be admitted to a respite bed available for the terminally ill, where in the early hours of the morning she died. Unfortunately, the previous day her brother had died suddenly and it was felt that the news had contributed to her 'giving up'. Her husband was revisited by the GP and admitted to hospital. He was then transferred to a renal unit with acute renal failure.

The nursing team felt very angry at the GP's decisions regarding the whole situation. They felt that they were unable to offer the standard of care that the couple needed due to the stubbornness of the GP. It left the nurses feeling very subdued and at a loss as to what to do. They also felt inadequate in their role. On questioning, the GP was surprised at the events but still stated that the lady could have lived until Christmas. Unfortunately she didn't'.

Case study 5.1 Critical incident: dysfunctional multi-disciplinary team work

The realities of practice are clearly illuminated through this critical incident, and the potential to learn from this through adopting a reflective approach is enormous. The incident described in case study 5.1 provided the focus for discussion with the student and the mentor during a practice placement visit, as well as with a group of student district nurses during a session exploring critical incidents. Many of the issues raised in other incidents were similar.

The incident was explored using the experiential learning cycle model as a framework for analysis (Smith & Russell 1991, 1993). After sharing the incident with me the student and mentor described how the incident had left them feeling angry, frustrated and at a loss as to what to do. This is clearly evident in the student's account of the incident, where some of the terminology is very emotive. The initial discussion centred on possible explanations for this incident, from a variety of perspectives. (It is important when using an incident of this nature to be as objective as possible, avoiding a moaning session; to use it as a basis for developing practice, not as a technique to apportion blame.) This was followed by an exploration of both formal and informal theories, which helped the student and mentor begin to shed light on the experience as well as begin to consider how they could address some of the issues raised both now and in the future.

It would be impossible in a chapter of this length to provide a detailed account of the discussion and emergent issues; what follows is a flavour of some of the points raised, together with some of the literature referred to.

The discussion commenced with the feelings of lack of control and the powerlessness experienced by the student and mentor. Issues such as professional power, disempowerment (Foucoult 1983), perception of control and its relationship to stress were raised and explored in an attempt to understand the incident (Parkes 1984). This led into an analysis of the functioning of the primary health care team, discussion of awareness of each other's roles, role boundaries, and multi-disciplinary working (Hudson *et al.* 1997; West &

Poulton 1997b; DoH 1998g). This was linked back to perceptions of professional power and the role of the specialist practitioner.

Exploration of patient and carer rights then emerged. This was located in the policy context exploring concepts such as choice, patient empowerment, patient advocacy, and the provision of a needs-led service and issues of unmet need (DoH 1989b; Morriss 1994; Arber & Ginn 1995; Ungerson 1997). We then moved on to discuss grief and loss as the death of the lady's brother was seen as a contributing factor in her 'giving up'. It was at this point that the mentor began to describe some of the characteristics of a rural community, particularly the fierce independence evident among some of the older members of the community who were often reluctant to accept help.

The importance of evidence-based practice was discussed at length and was seen as a vehicle for questioning the GP's decision-making (Trinder & Reynolds 2000). However, both the student and mentor acknowledged that they needed to review and develop communication channels between the GP and practice team as well as develop their own assertiveness skills. They also discussed how they would raise with their line managers the issue of the unmet needs that were evident, the intention being to explore referral processes and configurations of services in an attempt to prevent a similar situation occurring. The practitioners involved had clearly moved through an experiential learning cycle from describing and attempting to explain the situation to consideration of current and future actions (Smith & Russell 1991, 1993).

Reflection on process

It is clear from the analysis that we were drawing on knowledge from a variety of disciplines such as psychology, sociology, social policy and nursing as well as knowledge that the practitioner had acquired through working for many years in a rural community. I must however reiterate that the references cited are *examples* of the type of material drawn upon to inform the discussion and critical discourse. When this incident was analysed with a group of district nursing students, almost identical issues were raised. It must however be noted that due to time constraints in the classroom many of these were covered very superficially, with the teacher providing prompts. This is where the relationship between the use of a reflective framework and problem-based learning (enquiry-based learning) becomes evident. Clearly, in an hour's supervisory session, a short placement visit or a three-hour workshop in the classroom, it is impossible to explore all of the issues raised in depth. Students are rarely able to discuss theories in detail, let alone critically appraise their value in enhancing understanding of practice, unless they have recently explored them in the classroom or through an academic or practice-based assignment.

Problem-based learning offers a possible way around this. This is a method of learning which encourages students to work in small groups to gather knowledge and develop problem-solving skills (Wilkie 2000). With this approach real life problems are presented to the student who then has to gather knowledge relevant to the context. Wilkie (2000, p. 11) cites Howard Barrows, who described problem-based learning as a 'closed loop' process of 'encountering the problem first, problem solving with clinical reasoning skill and identifying learning needs, self study, applying newly gained knowledge to the problem and summarising what has been learned'.

There are clearly some similarities between using a reflective cycle to analyse practice scenarios and problem-based learning. For example, the starting point for both is an issue from practice. The next stage in the reflective cycle goes on to ask what has happened and how can it be explained through reference to both formal and informal theories. Similarly, problem-based learning asks what learning needs to take place to solve the problem. Students are then directed to learn that which is appropriate. Each student independently explores a different aspect of learning prior to feeding back to the main group. It is this stage of negotiated learning that I am arguing needs to be made more explicit when undertaking critical incident analysis, otherwise we may be at risk from making assumptions about the students' knowledge base.

This can be achieved in both the classroom and in practice through building in time to enable the student(s) to explore knowledge underpinning practice in greater depth. It may be worthwhile for mentors to consider meeting with groups of students in the locality to develop this technique. This could serve to reduce the amount of work that each student needed to undertake as well as provide a means of support for both students and mentors. This stage is relatively easy to incorporate into classroom activity through follow-up workshops. The process can also be encouraged on an individual basis through the use of a learning diary. Only when all of the gathered information has been considered can new learning of relevance to the practice scenario be identified and strategies to develop practice be considered and tested.

Critical incident analysis has proven to be very popular, with the following benefits identified through evaluations and discussion:

- Enabled students to further develop problem-solving skills
- Enabled students to develop skills in reflection
- Problems could be explored in a safe environment
- Use of the process clearly demonstrated the relationship (or otherwise) between theory and practice
- Helped to uncover practice-based knowledge
- Opportunities for practice development and the development of evidence-based practice became evident (See Chapter 7 for ENB Higher Award)
- Helped to develop confidence
- Could see potential of using the technique for clinical supervision sessions and with other staff in practice.

It is important to note that on a few occasions a student has become upset and has had to leave the group, particularly if the incident is 'too close to home'. It is therefore important to have some awareness of their needs as well as some support systems in place for the rare occasion they may be needed. Furthermore, mentors using this approach for the first time will need the support and guidance of a colleague with more experience in using the technique. As I said at the outset, reflection is a learned process.

Chapter 6

Clinical Supervision for the Specialist Practitioner Student

Peter Wilkin

Peter Wilkin is an authority on clinical supervision and provides here a chapter on his subject that is both detailed and poetic. The rationale for presenting a chapter on clinical supervision is that the inherent principles and concepts mirror the quality practice support that all students should expect of their mentor. For the uninitiated, this chapter provides background, theory and policy. The links between reflection and clinical supervision become evident as it progresses to a discussion of how educational clinical supervision works in practice.

Introduction

Over the last decade, the concept of clinical supervision in nursing has progressed from the isolated clarion calls of the early disciples to a number of established and evaluated systems throughout the UK (Butterworth & Woods 1998). It has gained popularity as 'a formal process of professional support and learning' (DoH 1993), although resistance from nurse practitioners and managers alike has been considerable (Wilkin *et al.*, 1997). Whilst the latter have clamoured for evidence of its cost effectiveness the nurses themselves have understandably verbalised their suspicions that supervision will be imposed on them as a covert means of surveillance (Castledine 1994). Nevertheless, despite such reservations, clinical supervision continues to play an important role in the individual support and development of nurses and as a method of quality assurance.

Owing to the diversity of disciplines and therapies that have adopted it as an integral part of their roles, definitions of supervision abound. In the nursing field, however, there does seem to be some correlation, in that supervision is seen as 'An exchange between practising professionals to enable the development of professional skills' (Butterworth 1998, p.12). Whilst Butterworth's definition provides us with the process and rationale of supervision, Power (1999, p.21) offers us a more comprehensive 'six-point plan' which contains both 'the purpose and direction of clinical supervision in nursing':

(1) Reflect upon the supervisee's practice
(2) Promote learning and advancement of skills

(3)   Be skills-based as its application
(4)   Be supportive of the supervisee and open to changing needs
(5)   Have the best interests of the patient as the highest priority
(6)   Encourage safe and independent practice.

Quite clearly, Power's blueprint reflects the essence of clinical supervision, which is the support and development of the nurse.

There is also corroborative evidence in virtually all the nursing literature (Bishop 1998, p.9) that clinical supervision contains a framework of three basic functions, initially defined from within social work circles by Kadushin (1992, pp.19–20). These are administrative (or managerial), educational and supportive, which cover all aspects of the supervisory process. The managerial component provides the quality control aspect of supervision, whilst the educational task is to promote the development of the specialist practitioner's skills and knowledge. The supportive function, as implied, provides a vehicle of response for nurses engaged in clinical practice who continuously find themselves being battered by such an emotionally demanding profession. From within her role as counselling trainer, Proctor (1991, p.62) identified three very similar strands which enabled her students to develop standards, skills and understanding within a safe and refreshing climate. She gave the much softer labels of normative, formative and restorative to her components. There is also much more of a sense of togetherness in Proctor's interpretation projected by her Winnicottian (see notes at the end of this chapter) references to the 'good-enough' learning environment. Teaming up with Francesca Inskipp in a later publication, Proctor describes the educational, or 'formative', task of supervision as being a 'shared responsibility for the (supervisee's) development in skill, knowledge and understanding' (Inskipp & Proctor, 1993, p.6). This sense of relationship facilitates the most rewarding engagements in any supervisory context.

Educational clinical supervision

Kadushin (1992, p.135), in the third edition of his seminal text, leaves us in no doubt as to the purpose of educational supervision: '[it] is concerned with teaching the worker what he needs to know in order to do his job and helping him to learn it'. His interpretation of educational supervision seems to be that it is predominantly role specific and an adjunct to the administrative component. At times, Kadushin's model of educational supervision falls into paradox, as andragogy and pedagogy seem to lock horns and stumble over each other. His andragogical intention of 'individualising' the learner is simultaneously abrogative and disempowering as he makes his 'educational diagnosis' (p.168) on each and every student.

The more general trend seems to be to celebrate clinical supervision as a whole package, with the emphasis firmly on clinical development and support. The educative or formative function is usually presented as a training exercise geared towards further learning in the shape of skills, knowledge and understanding. Much emphasis is placed on the supervisory relationship as a vehicle for learning, with the student's experiences providing the route markers. Indeed, many texts make only scant reference to the educative component by name, preferring to focus instead on the training process (Stoltenberg & Delworth 1987, pp.137–51) and the various stages of trainee competence (Hawkins & Shohet 1989, pp.48–53; Inskipp & Proctor 1995, pp.122–8).

Within the field of specialist practice, the topic of educational supervision is remote to say the least. In some ways, specialist students can be compared to trainee counsellors or therapists, in that they need to become good enough to practice within a designated period of time. Their practice placements in specific clinical areas provide them with their praxis opportunities. Every chunk of clinical practice presented in supervision, therefore, needs to be academically and organisationally contained: double-wrapped by curriculum content and corporate protocol. Yet, in other ways, specialist students are unique in that they already possess a qualification of nursing competence. Indeed, some students have already 'practised' in their particular speciality for a period of time without an official rite of passage. Such potentially vast variations in levels of individual experience need careful consideration and exploration by student and mentor at the beginning of (or even before) each practice placement. It should not be taken for granted that any first level nursing qualification carries a guarantee that the student knows how to 'be with' the 'other': either practically or interactively. Selected clinical case studies, therefore, need to feature frequently in the supervisory sessions.

Although each specialist student totes a pre-determined learning agenda, this should not in itself shape the supervisory process. Whilst it may direct the supervision contract and influence the content, the three functions of supervision remain inextricably linked and all will come into play during each and every session. Consequently, labelling such supervision 'educational' is misleading; all supervision should be educational in that all supervisees should leave the session having transcended their pre-sessional threshold of learning. There will be instances of restorative and normative processes in every supervision session and a purely educational session should never happen. This being so, the most appropriate description of such sessions seems to be clinical supervision, qualified through the phrase 'clinical supervision for specialist practitioner students'. All the usual boundaries and privileges of clinical supervision will also apply. Whilst prudence and context prevent a detailed explanation of how that translates, a summary of the main implications is provided purely as a launching pad for any further exploration. A detailed account of how to develop and introduce a system of clinical supervision is provided in Bond and Holland (1998, pp.216–28).

Prerequisites to clinical supervision

Mandate

When clinical supervision is to be introduced into any area of nursing, it is essential that the appropriate manager provides a mandate (Wilkin 1998a, p.200). Without this official 'permission to act', supervision could be interpreted as an optional exercise, which would reduce its credibility and effectiveness. Supervision without approved permission invites avoidance and may be taken away at any time. The clearest, most secure form of mandate is provided in the form of a written protocol, which includes a supportive statement from the organisation and a vision of the finished product.

Policy

Once a mandate is granted, all the stakeholders must be represented in the formation of a written supervision policy. Such a policy will outline the chosen system of supervision, together with the process and the boundaries involved.

Standards and audit

As supervision is implemented, standards need to be created to provide measurable baselines from which to identify performance levels, resource deficiencies and training needs. New systems of supervision need to be audited thoroughly and as soon as possible after the implementation date (Webb 1997). The data collected can then be used as a baseline from which the initial standards can be created. When audited on a regular basis, standards contribute significantly to the development of a quality system of supervision.

Contract

Creating a supervision contract encourages both supervisor and student to approach their supervisory relationship as partners (Wilkin 1998b, p.14). It also identifies the boundaries which separate supervision from the mentor's role of assessor. Both processes need containing within two separately negotiated contracts. Whilst presenting an opportunity to get to know each other better, the supervisory contract establishes some basic guidelines which contain the supervisory process and identify individual responsibilities. The most common contractual issues are time and frequency of sessions, confidentiality, documentation and evaluation.

Boundaries

Presentation boundaries also need to be constructed to determine the content of the supervision sessions. 'Clinical' supervision implies, quite clearly, that it is a practice-oriented process and, whatever the student brings to the session, it must in some way connect up to his clinical practice. If the student does bring material to supervision such as personal issues or inter-departmental conflicts, that is not to say that the mentor should immediately reject it without consideration. It is perhaps more prudent for her to listen for a few minutes until she is fairly confident that the presentation is inappropriate. A tentative intervention full of warmth and respect can then respond to the situation without it feeling dismissive.

If the incident being related is more of an expression of dissatisfaction towards another team member, for example, the supervisor's role would be to acknowledge what the student is saying (including the student's feelings) and then to make it clear that supervision is not the best forum to deal with this. It would be more appropriate to engage in some form of managerial supervision here: either with the mentor outside the supervision session (this may sound pedantic to some, but it does give a very important boundaries message to the student and it also protects the student from losing precious clinical supervision time through polluting it with inappropriate issues) or, perhaps, the team leader. If, on the other hand, the student has brought an issue such as a personal bereavement which is causing him immense distress, the mentor's response would be quite different. Whilst it is still important, at some stage, to declare that this is not clinical supervision, one of the best responses might be to abandon the session as a supervision session and agree to re-book it (so the student does not miss out). The allotted time can still be used as an opportunity for the student to talk about his distress – in other words, to officially turn it into supportive conversation. It may well be that the session becomes a valuable experience which the student was desperately in need of and, probably, a good opportunity for the mentor to suggest that time away from work might well be the student's best option.

Sometimes, students who have failed to grasp the rationale behind clinical supervision may renege on their responsibilities. For example, they may turn up late for sessions, attempt to end the session prematurely, or try to engage the supervisor in social chit-chat. Such instances are not to be pounced on by the supervisor in punitive fashion, otherwise the likelihood of an unproductive transference/counter-transference situation ensuing is high (see notes at the end of this chapter). Instead, the mentor needs to see such resistance as exciting opportunities for exploration and, of course, potential parallel processes full of unconscious information about the student's clinical encounters. But let us also stay real because there may be some quite simple explanations preventing the student from honouring the supervisory contract. She may be a single mother fighting to care and provide for her children and, consequently, struggling to fulfil all her commitments. The only acceptable response from the mentor under such circumstances is: 'Well, how about if we book an hour together as soon as possible to see if we can make some changes that might help you'.

The worst possible scenario which we must always dread is that the student's failure to engage in supervision is caused by a general lack of interest and motivation. If the supervisor suspects this to be the case, she has no option other than to gently but purposefully confront the student with both her suspicions and the evidence behind them. Failure to do so would represent a relinquishing of the mentor's responsibilities.

Power

Clinical supervision provides a stage on which power dances energetically throughout the whole performance. Given the nature of the designated roles within supervision, it is the supervisor who finds herself in a position of influence, able to sustain or restrain the student, often with just a few chosen words. On occasions, the clinical supervisor will pick up on a particular practice issue and guide the student's exploratory journey. Whilst navigational skills sit comfortably within the role of the supervisor, it is a cardinal sin to suddenly grab the helm. It is often much easier to offer solutions than to experience the frustration of watching the student stumbling around in the dark. Being in a position of nominated expert carries with it the temptation to provide answers instead of patiently sitting amidst a power failure of ideas. Good-enough supervision involves being with the student long enough until he, himself, finds the light switch.

The clinical supervisor's badge of office may well invite a variety of challenging behaviours from the student. Eager to please and impress his senior colleague (who will also have the responsibility of assessing his proficiency), he may attempt to curry her favour in a variety of ways. Whilst downright pleasantness is to be greatly encouraged, the student who tries too hard to please needs to be informed that this is unnecessary. Indeed, it should be made clear from the start that challenging his supervisor whenever necessary is the order of the day and that he will be thought all the better of for doing so. Clinical supervision is full of two-way conversation and the route towards shared understanding sometimes requires a thorough interrogation of the other's belief system. From within a framework of mutual respect, this can be a rewarding and enjoyable experience.

It is much harder to respond to a situation when the student takes umbrage at the supervisor's constructive criticism. On such occasions, the potentially difficult yet essential task of the supervisor is to confront this defensive behaviour. There is no acceptable justification for negatively reacting to the supervisor's challenges providing they are delivered caringly and tentatively. Under such circumstances, it may be that the student is carrying baggage and inappropriately displacing his feelings onto his supervisor (see notes at the end of the chapter).

Empowerment

From within a cluster of regulating and controlling frameworks (clinical governance, DoH legislation, local policies and protocols) emerges the mandate that authorises the construction of a vehicle of empowerment within a system of power. What has evolved is a process we call clinical supervision, where the student brings along clinical material from his practice to discuss with the supervisor. During the ensuing dialogue, the couple work together towards understanding things differently and more comprehensively. Conversation becomes the grid from which power is able to flow. The student (and the supervisor) knows more and can use this extra knowledge to determine future practice. He has been empowered through the betweenness of the supervisory relationship (Wilkin, 1999).

Kadushin (1992, pp.78–134) covers this contentious subject thoroughly and advocates openness on behalf of the supervisor who 'must accept, without defensiveness, or apology, the authority and related power inherent in his position' (p.95). Only from within this open stance is the supervisor able to share her power and, consequently, empower the student. The relationship is both the place of conception and the birthing place of power (Crossley 1996, p.136). Acknowledging this and using the intersubjective space as a point of transfer for power, balances the supervisory relationship and serves to empower and sustain the student. Simply being there and resisting the urge to take control allows the student to become empowered through creatively searching for and eventually finding direction and understanding.

Kadushin (1992, p.87) also introduces the notion of referent power, where the student strives to be like the supervisor. Whilst such a state of affairs could be misused by the latter to disempower the former, it can also serve as a marker which motivates the student to reach the same high standards of practice achieved by his supervisor. As a result of such identification, the student may go on to internalise the supervisor's expectations and use them as a guiding light for his own practice.

Assessment and supervision

As both supervisor and assessor, the mentor's role is a potentially conflictive one. Supervision is an essentially non-judgemental process and a great deal of energy has been directed through various texts towards separating it from any surveillance exercise. The 'misleading and inappropriate name' debate has dragged on, now, for years as nurses and counsellors have objected to the panoptical implications of the word 'supervision' (Williams 1992). Perhaps this represents the general anxieties of nurses who feel unsafe and unprotected amidst an increasingly demanding work environment. Strange that psychotherapists do not seem to carry the same reservations, and revealing perhaps that medical practitioners have never adopted the term. Interesting, too, that nurses have not levelled the same argument against clinical governance, with its even more aggressive connotations.

Whilst labels do indeed conjure up particular images and elicit certain reactions, clinical supervision is a process designed to protect and enlighten; or, as Barker (1998, p.67) propounds, 'to protect people in care from nurses and to protect nurses from themselves'. All those who receive it in its intended form (offered, structured, and delivered by 'experts') are inevitably pleased with it. The situation need be no different in community practice education. Providing the mentor has received some credible training as a supervisor (and, even better, been on the receiving end herself) and is familiar with the rationale behind it, she should make it available as a regular feature for the specialist student.

However, clinical supervision does not carry with it any exemptions if codes of practice are seriously transgressed. In such instances confidentiality must be broken, otherwise, the concept of supervision becomes meaningless and valueless. By the same token, supervision provides the supervisor with countless opportunities to sustain, validate, praise and reward the student practitioner: an exercise that happens all too infrequently within nursing in general. Nurses are valuable and special; it makes sense to treat them as such. Genuinely positive responses help to reinforce this: 'You've really engaged Jenny, haven't you? It sounds as though she's really reaping the rewards of your interventions ... that's great'.

Training

If clinical supervision is to become an integral part of specialist student education, it should be provided from within a framework that guarantees consistency and comprehensiveness. Although the students represent a variety of disciplines, the supervisory format should contain certain boundaries and opportunities that are relevant to all specialties. Such systems can be created and inserted into the curricula of the specialist student (with the emphasis placed on how to be a supervisee) and the mentor (with the accent directed towards the supervisor).

The supervisory relationship

It is within the supervisory relationship that the student needs to feel safe enough to pour out her feelings. The experience of being safely contained is an intimate affair. It is 'a communion with otherness' (Crossley 1996, p.28) that happens within the space between two people. Rather than an exchange of words involving two separate people, it is a joining together through a shared language. Yet, strangely, there is usually a third person (and sometimes many more) present within the room who, on occasions, make the fusing of individual horizons nigh on impossible. Whilst student and supervisor sit together consciously aware only of each other, unconscious fantasies and processes infiltrate into and pollute the conversation. Supervision becomes a house haunted by ghosts from past life experiences, some of them only hours old and others which are rooted in the dim and distant past.

Tilly was a student occupational health nurse in the middle of presenting her client, Marjorie. As her supervisor, I became aware that my attention had drifted momentarily and I quickly made a conscious effort to tune in once more. This was quite strange, as Tilly was quite an animated and enthusiastic supervisee who positively grabbed my attention with her breezy presentations. Yet I had become detached and an empty feeling had momentarily engulfed me. I decided to share my uncharacteristic departure with Tilly and explained to her that I had found myself drifting, feeling quite empty. 'I wonder if that means anything to you at the moment?', I tentatively enquired. 'Well, I guess that's just how Marjorie explains the way she feels,' Tilly responded. 'Cut off and empty.'

We pursued these two metaphors and followed the trail back to the comprehensive history that Tilly had taken from Marjorie. And there lay the possible link: Marjorie had undergone a hysterectomy 18 months ago at the age of 37. Shortly afterwards, her mother had died after suffering her second cerebro-vascular accident. Both Tilly and Marjorie had focused on the inevitable loss issues brought about by this important bereavement, identifying this as the source of the latter's depression. They had 'packaged' the hysterectomy as both a positive intervention and 'over and done with'.

Following the supervision session, Tilly waited her moment during her next planned session with Marjorie and, when the time felt right, reintroduced the hysterectomy. It will probably come as no surprise to you by now that, by focusing more on feelings and the symbolism of such a drastic and invasive surgical procedure, the primary cause of Marjorie's depression turned out to be the loss of her reproductive capabilities. She disclosed that she had felt 'neutered' and, despite her hormone replacement therapy and a dramatic improvement in her physical health, her sexual relationship with her partner had gradually come to a standstill (which she had initially interpreted as part of the depressive reaction to her mother's death). Sensibly, after discussing all the options, Tilly referred Marjorie on to the Trust's counselling service. After ten sessions, Marjorie had worked through the grief of losing her 'womanliness' and re-engaged in a sexual relationship with her partner.

Case study 6.1 Counter-transference in clinical supervision

The narrative in case study 6.1. highlights the potential power contained within the supervisor's raw counter-transference feelings. My shared sentence that, initially, made virtually no sense to me was the spark that ignited Marjorie's road to recovery. The content of both transference and counter-transference reactions can be interpreted to provide insight for the student practitioner into both himself and his clients (Hawkins & Shohet 1989, p.64). Of crucial importance here is that the mentor understands the phenomenon enough to interpret it safely and productively. Clinical supervision for the specialist student bears little resemblance to either psychotherapy or psychotherapy supervision. Any personal insights gained are valuable but supervision for the specialist student is geared towards ensuring that he becomes a competent practitioner before he is awarded specialist practitioner status. Consequently, all transference interpretations should be guided towards the practice arena as early as possible. Otherwise, boundaries may collapse and the supervision sessions mutate into personal therapy – a potentially damaging and completely unacceptable situation under any circumstances (Yegdich 1998, 1999).

Turning lived experience into learning experience

The process of all supervision is circular and perpetual. It begins at a point when supervisor and supervisee embark on an exploratory journey together. It is an expedition with no predetermined stations other than the end point of the supervisory session. Eventually we return to the starting point, which now becomes the finishing point, as we put together all the parts of the journey to make a whole: a new way of seeing the practice incident in the light of all that has transpired within the session. From every session of supervision there is always a narrative which was that session and which now reflects that session. This supervisory story will, hopefully, contain chronological evidence of a developmental journey, from the point of ignition (the issue that has been brought to supervision) to the vantage point at the summit of the whole experience. Looking back, the student can now see how his lived experience has slowly evolved and become a true learning experience.

A similar process forms the basis of all reflective practice: firstly, we have the experience; secondly, we return to that experience in order to reflect upon it; thirdly we re-evaluate the experience and integrate it into our conceptual framework; and, finally, we apply this newly formulated perspective as we encounter future situations which are similar enough to the original experience (Boud *et al.* 1985, p.18–40).

A reflective model of educational supervision

Supervision for the specialist student is neither a complicated nor an abstruse process. It involves a bout of facilitated reflection which focuses on clinical practice and enables the student 'to make sense of the mysteries of community practice' (Canham 1998). In order to ensure a productive supervisory journey, there need to be some identifiable structures which guide the supervisory couple down the scenic routes. Whilst this may seem like a poor choice of metaphor, there is little to be gained from taking the fastest route. You are likely to miss a great deal if you always stick to the motorways (besides becoming incredibly bored). Taking the scenic route along the tall hedgerows and winding coastlines is much more stimulating and exciting. There are many vantage points from which to view and plenty of hidden coves to explore. The experienced supervisor becomes a skilled navigator able to spot the potential beauty spots whilst, simultaneously, ensuring enough progress is made in the time allotted. Johns (1994) and others have shown that reflective practice is more productive when embraced by a structured framework. What follows is a brief guide for any reflective journey undertaken from within supervisory territory.

Casework moments

Before the supervision session begins, the student needs to identify a case-work moment: clinical experience for presentation. Rather than turning up to the session cold, it may be more fruitful if he has spent a little time reflecting on his experience and jotted down a few sentences or comments as a starting point. Casework moments come in various shapes and sizes. Generally speaking, they should contain a particular practice incident which the student feels the need to discuss.

Casework moments cover virtually every practice experience imaginable. If the student feels unable to identify a specific incident to present, he can choose to focus on a session that seemed relatively uneventful or that he felt went rather well. To believe that clinical supervision is unnecessary at any stage of a nurse's career 'because things are OK at the moment' is naïve to say the least. Every practitioner, whatever their developmental level, will always have blind spots and room for improvement in their practice. The skilled mentor should be able to isolate one single intervention – either comment or deed – and build at least one full session of clinical supervision around it.

The reflective scene is set, then, by describing the practice setting and the players involved. Whilst the major players usually turn out to be the student and his client, other players may emerge as key figures in the conversation, such as a relative, a doctor, a nurse colleague or a professional colleague from a different discipline. Once the cast has been identified the student can extract the issue for further exploration and, at the same time, share the reason for choosing this particular casework moment. Having allowed and encouraged her student to set his own supervisory agenda, the mentor's role becomes a mixture of courier, translator and agent of action.

Courier

Although the supervisory journey is a shared experience, the two travellers have distinct roles. The mentor often finds herself acting as a courier. Although she has never ventured down this particular route before, she has nevertheless encountered very similar terrain. She is aware of the potential pitfalls of such a journey and knows how to respond to just about anything they may encounter. She has prepared herself for all possibilities and the student rests comparatively safe in this knowledge. She will also ensure that the student does not miss any picturesque scenes or places of particular interest. She will keep the student well contained if they encounter dangers along the way. And she will be familiar enough with the route to ensure the journey finishes in time and ends at the right place. Collectively, she will be the student's experienced travelling companion, navigating when the pathways disappear and sustaining him whenever necessary.

Translator

During the student's practice placement he will encounter communications that defy interpretation and situations that do not make sense. Additionally, there will be clinical data that he misinterprets and even misses, which disappears into the ether as missed moments. Community practice can throw up situations that confuse the student and place him in a not-knowing situation. Such situations can trigger anxiety and feelings of hopelessness and frustration. The mentor's supervisory role here is not to find the answers or solve the problems. It is more to reframe the situations in a language that makes sense to the student, to wipe away the condensation that clouds his vision.

Agent of action

The reflective process, whilst circular, is inevitably progressive. Whilst the early stages of the supervision session will be filled with historical and exploratory past and present statements, the later stages will start to address future practice. During this later stage the reflective cycle is nearing full turn and reflection begins to succumb to projection. It is now that the mentor's interventions become more scripted, as she tries to ensure that the student has turned his lived, practical experience into a learning experience. This involves looking upstream to the next practice situation and identifying if he needs to practise differently, the ways in which he can do so and the possible consequences of doing so. As it nears its end, the supervisory journey should always be summarised and pulled together, with any identified objectives clearly stated. The mentor now becomes an agent of action, as she encourages the student to carry his learning experiences forward into the field of clinical practice. Finally, the student can leave supervision and transfer the essence of the session into his reflective journal.

Supervision for the mentor

The mentor needs her own supervisory forum in which she can discuss her clinical practice. Whilst she should undoubtedly be functioning at a higher developmental level than her student, she will still suffer from her own blind spots and, at times, need the support and containment that supervision has to offer. As Mander (1997) illustrates, the supervisor is always susceptible to the temptations of 'intellectual analysis' and her own 'preoccupations (and) narcissistic needs'. Within her role as mentor, she may also appreciate supervision sessions where she can share her supervisory experiences and tap into a system of support and development herself. Whilst a support group would serve some purpose, it would not carry a mandate to focus on supervisory interventions in any kind of critical or challenging way. Consequently, the mentor would not reap the benefits of being able to reflect on her supervisory practice in the company of a skilled supervisor. Perhaps time dictates that the most viable solution would be a mentor supervisory group – perhaps with three or four members – with either a revolving supervisor or a dedicated supervisor employed specifically within the role.

Envoi

The supervision session is not the place where we decide the outcome of our clinical interventions. It is, at best, a space in which, as supervisors, we can attempt to create the conditions of possibility for positive client impact. Within this creative space, our students bring us questions, incidents and dilemmas. Sometimes, we are tempted to provide answers and offer solutions to those problems, our weariness and complacency tempting us to fall into an arrogant frame of mind. On other occasions, we search for perfect responses to ideal situations, neither of which exist. As mentors we are ethically bound to introduce students to the world as it is, rather than as we might wish it to be. To act as though this world is other than it is would be unethical and mis-leading. It would remove opportunities to challenge and transform the world of practice and deny students 'their own future role in the body politic' (Arendt 1977, p.177). Clinical supervision provides the mentor with an opportunity to invite the student to reflect upon his practice and, in relation to that, ask the question 'who are you?' (Arendt 1958, p.178).

If the student arrives at the supervision session 'with mud all over his school uniform', the supervisor's response should be one of genuine accep-tance (Orlans & Edwards 1997). The field of community practice can be a veritable quagmire at times and muddy clothes tend to go hand in hand with such terrain. Berating the specialist student in any way, shape or form is a non-starter; it is guaranteed to encourage secrecy and defen-siveness. Indeed, falling over is inevitable (as the mentor surely knows) and, sometimes, leads on to the deepest level of learning. If the super-vision is 'good-enough', the student will avoid that particular practice pud-dle should he encounter it again. Rather than the mentor taking on the role of supervisory expert, it is the student and his practice that should take centre stage. Yet, despite these distinct roles, the wholeness of the supervisory process involves a journey of togetherness with no pre-determined route: a roam through the pathless woods that lead to each and every single nursing situation. The thing that is supervision exists within the interworld of the supervisory relationship. It involves the super-visor recognising and sustaining the student through a dialogue of shared understanding. The supervisor's quest is to make the student aware of just how creative he can be (Titchen & Binnie 1995). Clinical supervision is the intersubjective playground that should be built into the practice pla-cement of each and every specialist student.

Notes

It was Donald Winnicott, a respected paediatrician and psychoanalyst, who introduced the concept of the 'good-enough' mother into psychoanalytic theory. Rather than referring to the 'ideal' mother (which does not exist) he used the more realistic term of 'good-enough' to describe the mother (or primary parental figure) who was able to survive the child's challenging behaviour. Rather than becoming absorbed in feelings of inadequacy and guilt, the good-enough mother accepts the child's tantrums for what they are: immature expressions of fear and frustration. (See Winnicott, D. W. (1971) *Playing and Reality.* London: Tavistock.)

Transference is a psychoanalytic term which refers to the projection of certain characteristics or feelings which we have attributed to or experienced towards other people in the past, onto someone in the present. Whilst such a process is an inevitable part of ordinary life, it takes on a greater significance when clients unconsciously transfer their feelings, either negative or positive, onto the nurse or therapist. It is the supervisor's responsibility to confront the supervisee if the latter is unaware of or avoiding his client's transference reactions. Additionally, the supervisor is also susceptible to transference reactions from her supervisee. (See Chapter 6 in: Hawkins, P. & Shohet, R. (1989) *Supervision in the Helping Professions.* Buckingham: Open University Press.)

Counter transference reactions are the unconscious reactions to the initial transference reactions: either by the nurse to his client or the supervisor to her supervisee. In supervision, it is important that the supervisor remains vigilant for such counter-transference reactions which have emanated from the supervisee towards his client (and which have become apparent in the supervision session) or from the supervisor herself. Once recognised and understood, counter-transference can be a useful resource if used by the supervisor to provide reflective illumination for the supervisee.

Chapter 7

The English National Board Higher Award: A Strategy for Change

Joanne Bennett

The ENB Higher Award is presented here as an option to support the education of specialist practitioner students. Although it is not utilised by all HEIs, staff and students are enthusiastic about its benefits, particularly the focus on leadership and change. We are not sure what will happen to the Higher Award when the ENB (as we know it) disappears, but its principles (for example joint decision-making about an area for practice development) can be utilised by practice whether or not it is utilised as a formal method of learning.

Introduction

The complexity of professional practice and the changing demands placed upon community specialist practitioners to meet the requirements of their role and contemporary health care provision, are central themes in many of the chapters in this book. One of the mechanisms adopted at the University of Northumbria to introduce and prepare specialist practitioner students for this role has been the use of the ENB Higher Award framework. This framework has provided a useful structure to enable students to draw on knowledge gained through academic study and practice experience to lead and manage the process of change in practice. Although the ENB Higher Award is *not* an integral part of all specialist practitioner courses, and is *not* the only means of preparing specialist practitioners for their role as leaders and change agents, mentors may find the framework and process useful when facilitating the development of leadership skills at both the level of care management and at team level. I therefore intend to provide a step-by-step guide on how we have implemented this at the University of Northumbria at Newcastle (UNN), together with some of the benefits and challenges encountered.

What is the ENB Higher Award?

This is a professional qualification awarded to practitioners who are able to demonstrate mastery and integration of ten key characteristics into everyday practice (see Fig 7.1.) It may be awarded at either first degree or higher degree level. The Higher Award was developed out of recognition for those practitioners who wanted to continue to work in a practice setting and who wanted to undertake a course which was clinically relevant and which had practical application.

---

(1) The ability to exercise professional accountability and responsibility, reflected in the degree to which the practitioner uses professional skills, knowledge and expertise in changing environments, across professional boundaries, and in unfamiliar situations.

(2) Demonstrate specialist skills, knowledge and expertise in the practice area where working, including a deeper and broader understanding of client/patient health needs, within the context of changing health care provision.

(3) The ability to use research to plan, implement and evaluate concepts and strategies leading to improvements in care

(4) To demonstrate teamwork, including multi-professional team working, in which the leadership role changes in response to changing client needs, team leadership and team building skills to organise the delivery of care.

(5) The ability to develop and use flexible and innovative approaches to practice appropriate to the needs of the client/patient or group in line with the goals of the health service and employing authority.

(6) The ability to understand the use of health promotion and preventative policies and strategies

(7) The ability to facilitate and assess the professional and other development of all for whom responsible, including where appropriate learners, and to act as a role model of professional practice.

(8) The ability to take informed decisions about the allocation of resources for the benefit of the individual clients and the client group.

(9) The ability to evaluate the quality of care delivered as an on-going and cumulative process.

(10) The ability to facilitate, initiate, manage and evaluate change in practice and improve quality care.

Fig. 7.1   Characteristics of the ENB Higher Award (ENB 1991).

The decision to include the Higher Award in the BSc (Hons) Community Health Care Studies Course followed lengthy debate and the reasons for inclusion were numerous. First, when we compared the ten key characteristics of the Higher Award with the characteristics of specialist practice (UKCC 1994) we found a direct relationship between them. For example, the UKCC (1994) state the need for the specialist practitioner to 'demonstrate higher levels of clinical decision-making and be able to monitor and improve standards through supervision of practice, clinical audit, the provision of skilled professional leadership and the development of practice through research, teaching and the support of professional colleagues' (p. 9). (See Fig 7.1 for comparison). We therefore argued that students who fulfilled the criteria of specialist practice would *also* be fulfilling those of the Higher Award and should be given credit for this. Second, we wanted students to demonstrate the relationship between theory and practice (and vice versa), the process of the Higher Award being one means of achieving this. Third, we needed evidence that students were able to respond to and manage change in practice. Finally, we needed to ensure that students were equipped with skills in life-long learning. As we had already had success in using this framework with other post-registration nursing courses at UNN, it was our choice to continue to use this approach as one of the ways to facilitate the development of leadership skills and skills in change management.

While we recognise that the ENB Higher Award is implemented in different ways in other universities which have chosen to utilise the framework, we have adopted a learning contract to implement a change in practice. This contract is dependent on the student, the mentor and the university teacher working in partnership to support the student through the change process. Mastery of each of the key characteristics of the Higher Award is demonstrated during the process of change. Positive feedback about this has been received from graduates from the course (see Chapter 18), mentors, service managers and academic staff. However, recognition must also be given to some of the challenges posed when adopting such a strategy. Prior to considering these issues in greater depth it may be of value to offer some insight into how the process works in practice.

The process

The Higher Award encourages the student to adopt a systematic process to develop and/or change an area of their specialist practice. The process commences with a meeting between the student, the mentor and the university teacher to complete a tripartite contract. At this meeting ideas for the Higher Award are generated and discussed. The student is not required to make a firm decision at this point in the process. By the end of the meeting the three parties complete a tripartite contract where each person's role is identified. Examples of this are outlined in Fig 7.2.

Following this initial meeting there are four other Higher Award meetings.

First meeting – what to do (assess)

The first meeting is to decide on an area for development based on an *identified* need. It is therefore essential that the change identified is more than simply an area of interest to the student. This need may emerge from reflecting on the findings of the community profile which students must undertake and/or a critical incident (see Chapter 5). Further evidence required to justify the change is discussed and debated so that the student can collate this in preparation for the next meeting. Examples may include:

- Data from the health needs assessment
- Audit data from practice
- Evidence of local HImP priorities
- Analysis of critical incidents from practice
- Themes from a literature review
- Reference to local and national priorities.

The student role is to:

- Identify an area of innovation, implement and manage the change process
- Co-ordinate meetings between the student, mentor and university teacher
- Keep the contract up to date through recording key points from the discussion at the meetings
- Collect documentary evidence in relation to the innovation.

The mentor's role is to:

- Support the student in the selection of the innovation
- Assist with the provision of background information to support the need for change
- Act as a resource and a gatekeeper with other professionals who may assist with the change.

The university teacher's role is to:

- Provide advice on the completion of the contract
- Provide advice on the selection of the innovation to ensure that it is manageable in the time allowed
- Review the contract and the documentary evidence.

Fig. 7.2   Tripartite contract.

Second meeting – how to do it (plan)

At the second meeting the information, which has been collated to justify the change, is presented by the student and critically discussed by the team. For example:

- The strengths and limitations of the literature and research in the area of the proposed change are debated
- The relationship of the change to national and local policy is discussed, and the risks of the proposed innovation assessed
- Audit data from the practice is analysed.

Once it has been agreed that the change is justifiable in the light of the evidence, objectives are set for the next period. These objectives relate to the planning of how the student will take this innovation forward and the evidence required for the next meeting. Areas of consideration include:

- The consultation process e.g. managers, the trust, specialist nurses
- The group who will be directly involved, e.g. the immediate team, service users, representatives from other disciplines if appropriate
- The cost implications/resources
- The educational needs of those involved
- The methods of evaluation/monitoring
- The change strategy
- The time scale.

This information (and more) will be developed into a detailed action plan.

Third meeting – do it (implement)

The information collected since the second meeting is presented by the student and discussed. This may include:

- An action plan to take the innovation forward
- Minutes of meetings where views of colleagues have been sought
- Draft tools/designed documentation/leaflets etc.

Objectives, which relate to the implementation of the innovation, will be set and the evidence required identified.

Fourth meeting – how did it go? (evaluate)

At the final meeting the evidence collected will be reviewed. Students will be expected to review the *process* of initiating and managing change. Issues of consideration include:

- The personal learning which has resulted from undertaking the process
- The benefits to service users and colleagues
- The limitations/challenges posed during the process
- Areas for further development
- How they would do it differently if they were starting over again
- How they can share experiences with other colleagues.

Throughout the process, achievement of the key characteristics of the Higher Award is monitored. Students are expected to provide evidence of how these have been met; they are *not* expected to evaluate the impact of the innovation, as it is far too soon. Consideration is, however, given to how it could be evaluated in the future.

Over the past four years we have witnessed hundreds of innovative projects which have led to improvements in practice and have been continued, and in some cases, further developed by practitioners permanently located in that practice. Listed in Fig. 7.3 are a few of the innovations made by students when undertaking preparation for their role as a specialist practitioner.

In a chapter of this nature it is impossible to do justice to the true value of the Higher Award. What follows is an example of some of the issues

---

- The development and implementation of a positive parenting programme during the ante-natal period
- Raising awareness of accident prevention in pre-school children
- Health promotion events to meet the needs of young men
- The introduction of a system for the screening and management of hypertension
- The development of a communication strategy from the community to the acute sector
- The development of a nutritional assessment tool for use with the elderly
- The development of an assessment tool to identify those at risk from developing a leg ulcer, together with an outline protocol
- The development of a health promotion strategy to prevent iron deficiency anaemia during weaning
- The introduction of a sleep support initiative
- The development of an information leaflet – Healthy Backs Before and After Pregnancy
- Coronary heart disease – exercise referral for home base or leisure centre.

Fig. 7.3 Innovations in practice.

addressed by a student health visitor when attempting to empower mothers/ carers to weigh their own babies.

The idea emerged from the student reflecting on practice, and through the findings of the health needs assessment in the practice area. The student's placement area was a small village location in a rural area of north-east England. The area was extremely deprived, with above average rates of unemployment. Furthermore, the health needs assessment revealed a high percentage of under-fives in this village. It was also revealed that the population had literacy levels that were well below average, which was a particular consideration given the proposed innovation.

The student noticed that the baby clinics were extremely well attended, with many of the mothers using this as an opportunity to gather socially. The health visitor weighed the babies and general advice was given in the middle of a busy clinic. Many of the mothers 'hung back' after the clinics to try and have a private word with the health visitor, or if there was insufficient time, which was more often than not, to arrange a home visit. The student was concerned about the set-up at this clinic for a number of reasons, which she shared with her mentor and university teacher:

(1) The clinic appeared disorganised and was not meeting the mothers' needs in terms of offering opportunities for advice in private
(2) The skills of the nursery nurse were not being utilised to their full potential – she was 'assisting' the health visitor in the weighing of babies
(3) The mothers were not being encouraged to be involved in the weighing of their own babies – the health professionals were 'taking over'

81

(4)   The health visitors were 'run off their feet' trying to cope with numbers attending the clinics

(5)   Babies were weighed regardless of whether this was actually necessary.

From this initial reflection, the student proposed that mothers could become more involved and the clinic could become more efficient if the following changes were made:

- The clinic was re-organised to maximise the use of skill mix and offer mothers the choice in taking a more active role in the clinic through offering them the choice as to whether they wanted more involvement in weighing their own babies.
- To use the nursery nurse to prepare and supervise mothers for this process. This would 'free up' the health visitor and enable her to offer individual appointments to mothers during clinic hours.
- To increase health promotion activity through structured group sessions.

Although this appeared to be a small change the issues which had to be addressed were fairly complex. The first meeting therefore consisted of sharing ideas around the innovation prior to identifying the evidence that would need to be collected in preparation for the next meeting to justify the proposed change. This involved the student reviewing and analysing evidence to support (or refute) the change in practice through:

- Conducting a literature search in areas such as empowerment, risk management, clinic management, health and safety in clinics, user involvement and accountability
- Reviewing Trust policies and protocols in this area
- Analysing clinic data and data from home visits stemming from clinic overflow
- Analysing data from the case-load and local population
- Drawing together evidence from critical incidents from practice
- Gathering the initial views of health visiting colleagues who would be directly affected
- Contacting colleagues in other areas (local and national) who had initiated similar changes.

In addition to this, consideration was given as to how the characteristics of the Higher Award could be addressed should the change be justified.

At the second meeting the information and evidence that had been gathered by the student was shared with the mentor and university teacher. The strengths and limitations of the findings were debated. From the evidence it was agreed that the changes suggested by the student could be of potential benefit to the service user, practitioners and the organisation. However, the scale of the change was too extensive for the student to achieve in the limited time available. The mentor and the university teacher therefore negotiated with the student and the health visiting team that the student would be responsible for exploring issues around empowering mothers to weigh their own babies and other members of the team would take responsibility for other aspects of the change. It was however agreed that the student would take responsibility for the co-ordination of the project. The objectives and actions to be taken prior to the next meeting were then set. This involved the student:

- Consulting and obtaining the views of a wider audience, e.g. service users, other health visitors in the locality, GPs, local management
- Determining, with others, how and when the changes would take place
- Identifying and considering the preparation and development needs of colleagues and mothers and how these needs could be met
- Considering possible strategies that could be used to evaluate the impact of the change on service users, practitioners and the organisation.

This, and more, had to be developed into a detailed action plan to be presented at the next meeting.

At the third meeting the student presented a detailed action plan, together with evidence of any activities which had taken place since the previous meeting. This included:

- Lesson plans from when the idea had been presented to other groups
- Notes from any meetings
- Letters of correspondence
- Reflection of visits to other practice areas
- Personal diary entries.

Again the Higher Award characteristics that had been achieved were recorded. Further objectives relating to the implementation stage were then set, together with a follow-up date.

At the final meeting the student reviewed the process of change and considered how the project could be further developed, as well as the personal learning that had resulted. This included:

- The student highlighting some of the challenges and benefits of working through the change process in a structured and supported way
- The value (or otherwise) of using a reflective framework
- The challenges of involving service users and the need to ensure the mothers had a choice
- Strategies that she had used to facilitate the development of the nursery nurse, and the strengths and limitations of these
- The relationship between theory and practice
- The need to audit home visits and clinic appointments to begin to determine the effectiveness and efficiency of the change
- The need to evaluate the project from a service user's perspective, and how this might be achieved
- The need to evaluate the project in relation to staff satisfaction.

Although it was inappropriate to evaluate the project during the time span of the course, initial discussions and reflections with both staff and service users were extremely positive. Perhaps of more importance, the student felt well prepared to lead, initiate and manage change in practice and to do this from an evidence base. Chapter 18 provides a student's perspective of this process.

Issues for consideration

Following initial apprehension, the Higher Award has proven to be very popular with students, service colleagues, mentors and academic staff. This has been reflected in course and placement evaluations as well as through one-to-one discussions. One of the greatest benefits is that students, mentors and university teachers truly work in partnership to improve practice for the benefit of the service user. The environment in which the change takes place is a 'safe' place for the student as they are guided and supported through the entire process. The process facilitates skills in reflection, problem solving, workload management, teamwork, communication, enquiry-based learning, the development of evidence-based practice, and initiating and managing change (to name but a few). Furthermore, the students must clearly demonstrate the integration of theory to practice, and vice versa, through this process. In some instances the students have begun the process of articulating knowledge embedded in practice. Although we acknowledge that this is not the only strategy used to prepare specialist practitioners for their role, and that the lifespan of the ENB Higher Award is tenuous, we have found the process extremely beneficial.

The main drawback of this process is that it is time consuming. Each visit to practice may last between two and three hours. With student numbers for specialist practitioner preparation being in the region of 70–80 in any academic year, considerable demands are placed on limited numbers of academic staff with expertise in the area. Furthermore, time must be invested in the preparation of both mentors and university teachers prior to embarking on this process. However, the benefits to all parties far outweigh the limitations. As time has progressed, the trust and respect between mentors and university teachers has grown, these perhaps being some of the most important ingredients necessary when preparing future practitioners for the changing world of community practice.

Chapter 8

Assessment of Specialist Community Practice

Judith Canham

Assessment is an issue of concern to all teachers. New teachers, in both HEI and practice, invariably experience great anxiety about whether they are doing justice to the student. We consider this anxiety a healthy state of affairs, as complacency about the assessment of professional performance equates with complacency about practice.

In this chapter, Judith Canham concentrates on the issue of practice assessment and provides a series of examples that show how mentors assess students, and the dilemmas that can confront the unwary. To complement the 'common' principles of practice assessment we provide two HEI proformas for assessment: marking (grading) practice and the use of port-folios. Mentors reading this text may have experience of both or neither proformas but as in all chapters, the important issues are the applied prin-ciples.

Introduction

The issues, concerns, debates and dilemmas related to the assessment of practice are legion, and before exploring these points, it is worth stating that a perfect way of assessing practice may never be found (Jinks & Morrison 1997). The assessment of practice is far more complex than the assessment of an essay, and the higher the academic level the more difficult the assessment of practice becomes. Complicating the issue is the disparate nature of practice and the individuality of both students and mentors. Although students may be studying the same course, their individual learning needs, the student-mentor relationship and the learning environment are unique; the art of mentoring includes ensuring that practice assessment demonstrates equality and rea-sonable parity for all students undertaking a particular course. In other words, the assessment of each student must be comparable in terms of offered opportunities, quality and depth.

This chapter attempts to make sense of assessment in practice and offers mentors the opportunity for critical debate. An overview of the purposes and relevant methods of assessment precedes particular issues that mentors may confront. Case studies are provided to illuminate how mentors (and students) address the assessment process. Finally, there are two examples of the assessment of practice from higher education institutes: a strategy for marking practice, and the use of a portfolio.

Standards of assessment

ENB regulations (ENB 1995 p.91) require (all) assessment to:

- Reflect the inter-disciplinary nature of professional knowledge to achieve learning outcomes relating to theory and practice
- Reflect the principles of integration and coherence which facilitate learning
- Contain descriptors which help to discriminate between performance at differing academic and professional levels
- Provide regular and constructive feedback
- Assess theory and practice on an equal basis.

This regulatory framework provides the mentor with the basic 'rules' of assessment. Assessment should:

- Reflect multi-agency work
- Reflect integration of a variety of subject matter
- Contain evidence of achievements
- Provide feedback to students
- Be on a par with theoretical assessments.

This is all easier said than done. For example, to date there is no agreed strategy for describing performance at different academic levels (diploma, degree, postgraduate) and very few HEIs ascribe the same value to practice and theory assessment.

The integrity of practice assessment is enhanced when the mentor is fully integrated as a member of the course team at the HEI. In order to undertake any assessment of a student, the mentor needs to be fully aware of all parts of the curriculum and utilise this knowledge within the teaching, learning and assessment process as assessment is part and parcel of the entire learning experience (Quinn 1995). In other words, the question 'what theory is the student general practice nurse studying at the moment?' can identify the focus of learning for practice and the expected range of practice-focused knowledge.

Course curricula are based on UKCC (1994) and ENB (1995) outcomes that should be achieved by specialist students and it is this direction that provides the foundation for the assessment of practice. If the assessment of practice is underpinned by the course curriculum it should be fair, timely and related to prescribed UKCC and ENB outcomes; if assessment is based on the subjective expectations and experiences of the mentor it will be neither equitable nor consensual (Wong & Wong 1987). Providing students have been treated fairly by the assessment process, the professional judgement of mentors will not be questioned, but as in clinical practice, professional judgement may be considered insubstantial unless supported by an up-to-date knowledge base.

Purpose of assessment

The overall aim of assessment is to provide information that appropriate skills, knowledge and attitudes have been acquired (Somers-Smith & Race 1997) or, 'whether or not competencies have been acquired' (Quinn 1995). The assessment of specialist practice informs the HEI, the ENB, the UKCC, the public and prospective employers that the student has or has not achieved the outcomes of the specialist practitioner award. There is no doubt that this responsibility is onerous as the prospect of getting it wrong is not something that can be contemplated. The assessment of specialist practice is a complex process that takes time, energy and commitment (Jinks & Morrison 1997) and to enter mentoring is to enter the complicated world of practice assessment.

Most importantly, the assessment of any nursing practice is to guarantee the care and the protection of clients (Somers-Smith & Race 1997). Although the protection of clients appears to be met through safe and competent practice, Jinks & Morrison (1997) and Quinn (1995) point out that this is not always adequate, as a student may provide safe client care but may not use appropriate interpersonal skills when working with patients. In other words, the nurse may be task-competent but fail to demonstrate the art of specialist practice and the meanings, intentions and reasoning that underpin actions, whether that be patient/client care or team leadership.

Types of assessment for specialist practice

Formative

One of the most important types of assessment for practice is the formative or developmental assessment (Quinn 1995). Its importance lies in its ability to provide feedback for further development and identify underachievement at an early stage. This type of assessment is related to enabling and development and is an opportunity for providing student feedback. For example:

> 'So far you seem to be progressing well in most aspects and you are at the level you should be for this stage in the course. However you need to take a greater leadership role function.'

Summative

The summative (or final) assessment is usually carried out at or near the end of a course. In the case of practice assessment, summative is the formal assessment that contains a statement by the mentor that will either support the student's practice competence or suggest that they are not yet competent at the specialist practitioner role.

Continuous

Continuous assessment is the most commonly used form of practice assessment in the UK but is only truly continuous where the student and assessor relationship is also continuous throughout a course of learning (Jarvis & Gibson 1985). It is thus evident that mentors of specialist community practitioner students belong to the very small group that actually practises continuous assessment. As its name implies, continuous assessment is carried out over a period of time and normally, simultaneously assesses a student's performance in relation to a number of learning outcomes. For example, the student's use of appropriate interpersonal skills and the student's ability to manage care, will be assessed by the mentor over a period of time and in various client situations. Unlike 'one-off' assessments, continuous assessment can accommodate observed 'errors' (i.e. of judgement) as long as the shortcoming is followed by professional development. When used in conjunction with formative assessment, continuous assessment encourages mature professional practice especially if the student takes an active reflective part in the process.

Jo is a community learning disability nurse (CLDN) student. Her student caseload includes working within homes managed by a private care agency. A number of her clients are incontinent of urine and are regularly prescribed 'pads'. Jo feels this is inappropriate and works with the home to educate formal carers and clients. Her mentor assesses Jo's progress early on (formative assessment) and notes 'during discussion Jo is keen to reduce pad usage and increase continence but seems to have little knowledge of the facts, demographic and symptomatic, that influence incontinence in the learning disabled population'. Jo's mentor meets with her immediately after the visit to practice and lets Jo describe her intentions and reasoning and then asks:

Is incontinence a major problem in CLD nursing?
I don't know exactly
Do you think that nurses/carers treat the LD population differently from the rest of the population?
I don't know but probably
OK. Are there any issues that are specific to the LD population?
Well yea. Perhaps because they don't expect as much from health care, they're not treated the same, they may have difficulty expressing themselves, their incontinence may be more difficult to treat, um . . .
OK. I think this is a very good area for practice development but you need to do some more work to convince me that you're operating at a specialist level. OK?

Jo was evidently applying appropriate and safe behavioural techniques but was not demonstrating the art of specialist practice: utilising knowledge, skills and attributes together to inform practice. Jo's mentor discussed her concerns with Jo, namely that Jo was intending to provide a good standard of care but that this was not yet adequate for a specialist practitioner. Jo needed to undertake private study (directed by the mentor) that investigated incontinence in the learning disabled population, the symptoms that could advise the nurse/formal carer, the training, background and educational needs of formal carers, and how the specialist practitioner should manage the care of learning disabled people within care homes. At this stage Jo's mentor reflected on why Jo had not undertaken the background research:

'I probably encouraged her but didn't inspire her at the appropriate level. Perhaps she was trying to show me how good she was by doing something that was tangible. Whatever, I evidently haven't got over to Jo what the role of the specialist practitioner entails. I need to draw her back from "doing" and get her into a critical thinking mode. This may be hard as she wants to "be doing things" and I'm going to have to say "hold on". I'll have to think about how to handle this.'

Case study 8.1 Continuous assessment: a means of enabling development

Assessment (as in the informal, formative style shown in case study 8.1) is used to provide feedback to both the student and the mentor and should be facilitative to ensure that the student is enabled to develop practice. Part of the responsibility for assessment is ensuring that the student has had the opportunity to learn (Chambers 1998). If the student has not been given feedback or provided with opportunities to develop practice, assessment may be considered to be unfair.

Having discussed her progress with her mentor, Jo felt embarrassed that she had attempted a change in practice without the appropriate knowledge and skills to back her actions. She also felt that if she was to be a specialist practitioner, she would need to delegate (at least) some of her intended care to another member of the CLDN team. Jo did her background reading and investigations, including speaking to the person responsible for funding continence aids. She then devised an interim plan for providing support and training to the formal carers in care homes. The care plan was to be instigated by other members of the CLDN team and she would retain overall responsibility. Jo discussed her plan with her mentor, who was then able to assess part of Jo's transition from first level nurse to specialist practitioner.

Assessment in practice is invariably on a continuous basis, as it is impossible not to continuously assess within a one-to-one situation. It is also regularly formative as feedback is provided on a regular basis. However, it also contains a formal summative approach as there is a need to finalise the process of assessment. Both mentor and student need to be absolutely clear about the type and method of assessment and how the process will be applied in practice.

Methods of assessment

Examinations, tests and essays

You may find that assessment and examination are sometimes used interchangeably, as to assess is to examine, but an examination in today's nurse education is either a seen or unseen essay question or multiple choice/short answer questions. Whatever the style of examination or test, the process will inevitably take place in a formal HEI setting under strict examination regulations and it is clear that this type of assessment has no place in the assessment of specialist practitioner students.

Invariably all specialist practitioner students will be required to write a series of essays that show the HEI that they have understood the taught aspects, have read widely and can write at the appropriate academic level. Additionally most specialist practitioner courses demand that essays *reflect* on practice and *integrate* theory and practice. Essay titles, and often a choice, are usually given to students at the beginning of a module and the student has to produce the final version 1–4 weeks after that module has been completed. Although essays are an excellent way of assessing the student's theoretical understanding of issues (i.e. palliative care), they simply demonstrate the student's ability to write about palliative care under controlled conditions but in no way demonstrate any competence to undertake palliative care in practice.

Initial (diagnostic) assessment

Undoubtedly this is one of the most important but understated methods of assessment for practice. It is undertaken at the very start of the placement and is an evaluation of the student's existing skills and strengths, their previous achievements and what skills, knowledge and attributes may be transferable to this new situation. The initial assessment provides the opportunity to identify learning needs and essential learning outcomes and agree how the teaching/learning process should be shaped. In short it is a profile of the student; how this profile influences the facilitation of learning is shown in case study 8.2.

Louise has been working as a nurse in general practice for three years. She had previously managed an out-patient department. Her most recent employment has been as the sole nurse in a single-handed GP practice. She has commenced general practice nursing (GPN) as a full-time student. All of the practice placement will be at her mentor's practice, a large GP practice with a team of three GPNs.

The aim of the initial joint assessment in the first week of placement was to complete a student profile and from that to identify Louise's learning needs. The profile identified that Louise's professional skills included cervical screening, asthma and diabetes. She had attended courses and her skills were certificated.

Louise was unsure about her learning needs as she felt that she was already competent at the role. She was undertaking the course to gain the specialist qualification and to complete her degree studies. At this stage, the mentor tactfully did not question Louise's competencies; however she did work through Life Long Learning (ENB 1995) with Louise, noting the difference between working in a specialist practice and being a specialist practitioner. At this initial assessment the areas for immediate learning and development were identified as:

- Working co-operatively as part of a general practice team
- Collaborative working with GPN colleagues
- Developing the knowledge and skills for the management of chronic obstructive pulmonary disease (COPD)
- Developing the knowledge and skills for the management of coronary heart disease (CHD)
- Underpinning all actions with relevant and contemporary research/ evidence.

As the mentor did not want to start the student-mentor relationship by 'testing' Louise's professional skills, she deliberately avoided putting Louise into situations where these skills would be used. Instead she decided to focus on the new learning needs. These were transferred into assessable learning outcomes so that after six weeks' exposure to practice, Louise would be formatively assessed on her ability to, for example:

- Critically discuss her understanding of the current management of COPD in general practice
- Identify how well current management of COPD meets the needs of the practice population
- Identify what skills, knowledge and attributes the GPN team requires to manage COPD
- Debate the value of a team approach to the management of COPD.

Simultaneously, other learning needs not clearly identified at the initial assessment will be teased out and clarified, so that Louise will be able to be assessed on other issues that originally she felt competent to undertake. For example, after 12 weeks' practice placement Louise may be expected to:

- Demonstrate the ability to manage the care of people with diabetes, using up-to-date research and evidence

- Formulate and defend an action plan for the development of the management of diabetes, utilising a multi-agency approach.

Case study 8.2 Diagnostic assessment: a starting point

Observation

Mark is undertaking the district nurse award, having already qualified as a health visitor. As his mentor presumed a good knowledge of community teamwork issues she was fairly laid back in relation to his work with colleagues. She was somewhat concerned to notice that Mark tended to work in isolation and rarely communicated with other members of the nursing team. At their next planned meeting she mentioned her concerns to Mark. He appeared irritated, not by what she said but by the fact that she had been observing his practice. Their discussion around this point included covert or overt observation, how it was possible not to observe, the level and content of the observation and when observation should become part of the assessment process. They agreed that Mark had been unrealistic in not expecting to be observed but that his mentor should have agreed the ground rules for assessment with him, early on in the practice placement.

Case study 8.3 Observation as an assessment tool

One of the most commonly used methods of assessment in all practices is the observation of a student's performance in real-life situations. Whereas observation is one of those skills that nurses are said to be good at, it should not be assumed that all nurses possess the skills necessary for fair student assessment by observation. In reality observation is an exceptionally complex method of assessment, demanding a deep understanding of possible behaviours that could be observed, explanation and interpretation of observed behaviours, and factors that influenced the observed event. The debate in case study 8.3 is not purely about what was observed but the process of observation as an assessment tool. In all cases of assessment it is essential for both parties to know why observation is important and what is being observed (Phillips *et al.*, 1993).

In case study 8.3 the mentor may observe Mark's ability to work collaboratively with all types of professional and lay people, looking for a level that promotes partnerships for the benefit of good care management. Additionally, the mentor may want to observe Mark actively seeking collaboration rather than just addressing it when he has to. Observation here may also include *listening* for negotiation skills in action and whether there is a degree of unwanted collusion. As in all other methods of assessment, if the student knows what is expected of them and has been provided with appropriate learning opportunities, then they have also been given the opportunity to succeed.

Other significant people (patients/clients, doctors and colleagues) will also observe the student and though this may be unintentional, they may communicate their positive or negative feedback to the mentor, who then has to determine the relevance and validity of these third party observations as the agenda of significant others is not necessarily in line with course outcomes for practice.

Critical discourse (discussion)

There can be little doubt that the student is subjected to considerable scrutiny from the beginning to end of the practice placement and this includes their ability to communicate acquired learning at a level commensurate with specialist practice. Critical discourse is a particularly useful method of assessment for specialist practice as the student can demonstrate their ability to interpret and critically evaluate both self and practice.

After their discussion about observation Mark's mentor asked him to reflect on the aims, benefits and constraints to team work in district nursing. Mark also agreed to try to increase his team participation over the next two weeks, after which time he and his mentor would meet to discuss his progress. That discussion (critical discourse) would be a formative assessment.

At the planned discussion, Mark took time firstly to illuminate his previous experiences where he was *the* health visitor, and the uncommunicative nature of his previous primary health care team. He then went on, unprompted, to reflect on his feelings of inadequacy when viewed against the skills of the district nursing team and how he felt he might be considered a nuisance. However, this wasn't simply a negative discussion and Mark continued to reflect whilst at the same time reviewing some of the material he'd recently been reading. Realising there were some gaps in his *articulated* knowledge, his mentor thought carefully before asking him questions as she didn't want this critical discourse to turn into a test:

> 'Mark. Do you think that the way in which this nursing team works is beneficial for the members of the team?' and: 'How do you think we could develop team work here so that it improves patient care?'

Case study 8.3 (cont.)

This discussion focuses on two issues: what has been learnt formally and what has been learnt through reflection on self and current practice. Through discourse the student is able to demonstrate their ability to think critically about issues that they may have previously taken for granted – in this case the purpose and intent of teamwork within district nursing.

Learning contract

In case studies 8.1. and 8.3 informal learning contracts were developed before planned, formative discussion. In educational terms a learning contract is an agreement between teacher and student (ENB 1996) that identifies what each party will do to meet a learning need (in case study 8.3 learning centred on team work), the time scale and how learning will be assessed. Learning contracts can also be formal and part of the course curriculum.

Chris is new to community mental health nursing (CMHN), and as a part-time student is still working as a staff nurse in forensic psychiatry. Chris and his mentor found that working diligently through the course and each module's aims allowed them to identify both his learning needs and areas for assessment. The course curriculum demanded that a practice learning contract be established as a basis for the assessment of practice. As Chris was still finding his feet he felt that being in control of the learning contract would help him to feel more aware of:

(1) What he already knew
(2) What he needed to learn and how
(3) His needs for teaching
(4) How he could chart his own progress
(5) When he should be assessed and how.

Chris would also keep reflective notes on the pleasures and pains of learning specialist practice in CMHN. Chris and his mentor agreed that despite other learning opportunities and occasions, they would meet at the end of each calendar month to assess formatively his progress through clinical supervision, focused on his educational needs and using both the learning contract and the reflective notes. They also agreed to be open and honest about Chris' progress and his satisfaction with the learning and teaching process.

Case study 8.4 A learning contract as a learning and assessment tool

Self-assessment

The learning contract in case study 8.4 can be seen to be both a teaching and learning tool and a method of assessment. In all aspects the student takes an active part and through reflection on practice experiences, undertakes a self-assessment of achievements. Whereas most traditional methods of assessment are 'teacher-centred', self-assessment does what it says it does, but it has been a relatively unpopular method of assessment in higher education. The arguments against its use tend to be situated in the context of reliability and validity. However, self-assessment is a valuable method to utilise within practice assessment as it allows the specialist student to accept responsibility for professional development, encourages critical appraisal of personal, professional practice and enables decision-making in relation to professional achievements. These strengths, acquired through participation in the assessment process, can later be transferred to clinical practice leadership when the student emerges as a neophyte specialist practitioner. Aside from the natural benefits to the practitioner, clients should also be advantaged by a professional carer able to think and work in terms of partnerships.

Reliability and validity

In theory, reliability means that the assessment should be able to be replicated and that the results of assessments applied over a period of time to different cohorts would show a high degree of consistency. Although potentially this would appear to be an insurmountable problem for specialist practice, a degree of consistency can be demonstrated in practice assessments when the assessment tool is broadly the same for all students and where mentors have the same interpretations of the practice application and expectations of assessment.

In relation to assessment, validity suggests that the assessment should measure what it says it does and match published outcomes. In this case the measurement would be the competency of the student to function as a neophyte specialist practitioner. One of the problems of the past was that mentors did not always assess in relation to a consensual measurement (course aims or ENB outcomes) but applied their own, subjective measurement of what constituted a good or not-so-good student practitioner.

It is fairly easy to see why practice assessment has hitherto failed to satisfy its assessors of its competence, validity and reliability. However Goding (1997a) feels that validity and reliability are inappropriate indicators of specialist practice and that they reduce practice to a list of objectives that bear little relation to the sheer complexity of practice:

'... community practice assessment is not an exact science, and at degree level, should be consistent with a creative, integrative interpretation of competence as a continuous process of development and deeper understanding.' (Goding 1997, p.160)

Identifying the academic level of practice assessment

When specialist practitioner education reached degree level, one of the problems faced by programme leaders was how to assess practice at that academic level. Gerrish *et al.* (1997) in a study commissioned by the ENB, found that the literature, course curricula and educators were generally unclear about the assessment of practice at different academic levels. There are many guidelines related to assessing written work at degree level, but generally these criteria have little to say about practice. For instance, a criteria for a level III/degree essay might be, 'Justifies argument based on an extensive range of literature' (ENB 1996, p.97).

It can be seen that while the ability to *justify* is an appropriate assessment indicator for level III as this relates to critical thinking, 'based on an extensive range of literature' is an inappropriate expectation for practice assessment. In reality the intellectual level of practice is exceptionally difficult to assess, though if learning outcomes (ENB 1995 and course curriculum) are met, these will generally be at a level consistent with degree studies. For example, if the assessment of practice focused on the student's ability 'to care', this would not be appropriate at the specialist level but if additional criteria were incorporated, the intellectual 'level' of practice can become apparent. Additional criteria that demonstrate 'care' competencies commensurate with level III may include:

- Manages the care
- Critically evaluates the care provided by self
- Monitors, critically evaluates and provides feedback to team members regarding care provided
- Enables care to be provided in a collaborative context
- Critically evaluates those factors that influence care provision
- Explores how care priorities are and should be agreed
- Interprets the decision-making processes in relation to care delivery
- Utilises relevant evidence, research and literature in the management of care.

It is important to reiterate that assessment criteria such as those noted above must be part of the teaching and learning process and not simply raised as points for assessment.

Practice assessment

Academia is not always comfortable with the assessment of practice (Chambers 1998; Wong & Wong 1987; Somer-Smith & Race 1997) as nursing practice is so difficult to classify in quantifiable terms; the more advanced practice becomes, the more difficult it is to capture what it is that is being assessed. Many practice assessment documents have failed practice in that the criteria neglect those issues that are so important to practice, for example the student's attitude (Quinn 1995). Many attempts and studies have addressed the assessment of practice (ENB 1996) and many authors write of the difficulties arising from the desire to assess practice 'properly' (Chambers 1998).

At the Manchester Metropolitan University (MMU), staff and specialist students felt that as the course was 50% practice and 50% theory, practice should have as much credence as theory and in reality that was not the case as practice was largely assessed through theoretical assessments. In order to partly redress the balance, a new system of assessing practice was devised, one that accredits specialist practice with 20 Level III credits. Although this is not perfect, as it should be 60 credits, it is a start. In order to accredit specialist practice, the new system includes a structured framework within which mentors from all eight specialist community practices have a degree of freedom to make professional judgements. A percentage mark is applied to the student's performance in practice as it stands during the very last week of the course. The lateness of the marked assessment allows those students who had been new to practice to catch up with their more experienced colleagues. Applying a precise mark to practice enables all parties to identify at what point the student is functioning before being allowed to re-enter the world as a specialist practitioner. A summarised version of this new assessment process follows.

The 'new' assessment of practice at the Manchester Metropolitan University (2000)

The assessment of practice has two elements. For the student it involves the completion of a practice learning portfolio that identifies learning though practice, evidence of achievements and reflection on the learning process. The mentor assesses through nine overarching practice assessment criteria, which act as benchmarks to ensure that in the context of specialist practice each student:

- Demonstrates competence in essential specialist practice skills
- Works co-operatively with colleagues, other professionals and lay workers
- Utilises a partnership approach with patients/clients/informal carers
- Shows professional sensitivity when working with patients, clients and informal carers
- Demonstrates appropriate inter-personal skills with patients/clients/ informal carers and other professionals
- Demonstrates knowledge of the professional, legal, ethical and moral implications of practice
- Regularly uses opportunities to teach and facilitate learning in a variety of situations
- Shows developing leadership skills in relation to clinical practice
- Clearly identifies personal life-long learning and continuing developmental needs.

Although the skills, knowledge and attributes are the same for each student, the exact content and the way that they will be applied in practice will vary dependent on both the student and the practice. For example, in practice assessment criteria 1, the clinical skills required of the health visitor student will be very different from those required of the occupational health nursing student, but the principle and spirit of assessment is the same.

Each of the nine practice assessment criteria has its own list of characteristics or criterion references that mentors use to articulate how they *know* the student has achieved that criterion. (The list of characteristics is too long to repeat here but includes such points as 'considers the financial implications of applied treatments'.) These assessment criteria are deliberately benchmarks rather than minimal achievements and each student is assessed three times against these criteria; two assessments are formative and one summative. All students are expected to improve as they progress through the course, and the developmental assessments are there to provide both the mentor and student with feedback:

- Are you meeting goals?
- What else do you need to do?
- Is there a need for student counselling?

The one summative assessment takes place in the last week of the course. It is based on the professional judgement of the mentor in relation to the practice assessment criteria, the student's self-assessment and mediation from the HEI. Here a mark is attached to the student's achievements as judged within the period of consolidated practice. (Mentors are prepared for applying marks to practice and are supported by the university teacher.)

It is hoped that over a period, this marked assessment of practice will establish its credibility through internal and external moderation and through the continued support of mentors and students. Some HEIs already have systems in place that apply 60 credits to practice (e.g. MacLellan 1996) and although MMU may seem overly cautious, we were also aware of the implications of practice assessment on the workload of the mentor.

Portfolio development *(Joanne Bennett)*

The development of evidence-based practice in nursing is gaining momentum with the establishment of centres for evidence-based nursing, such as that at the University of York, and the publication of evidence-based nursing journals. Indeed, specialist practitioner students are expected to develop portfolios of evidence to support practice competencies. They are required to base their decision-making in areas such as care management and clinical leadership on the best available evidence and to demonstrate this through the evidence collection that forms part of their portfolio.

Portfolio development as an integral part of community specialist practitioner preparation at the University of Northumbria

The introduction of portfolios into specialist practitioner courses has not been without its challenges. The evidence collated through the portfolio has to offer proof that the student has achieved their clinical competencies and, where appropriate, demonstrate that clinical decision-making has been based on 'best' available evidence. Despite students having critical appraisal skills prior to entry on the course, and undertaking further units in methods of enquiry as an integral part of specialist practitioner preparation, confusion about what constitutes the evidence base of nursing and the evidence base to the portfolio has tended to be at the forefront of any discussions with them. Furthermore, initial attempts at portfolio development by the students have varied considerably in terms of quality and quantity.

Our initial views, that we needed to be as flexible as possible and try not to be too prescriptive, soon became untenable. Whilst some of the students' portfolios demonstrated understanding of the process, with the evidence presented succinctly and appropriately, others lacked focus and the relationship of the evidence to either the clinical competence or clinical decision-making was questionable. It was at this point that we developed student guidelines for completion of the portfolio. Over a period of four years these guidelines have proven to be beneficial to students, mentors and university teachers and comments from external examiners reflect how the portfolios have become relevant and focused.

The following is some of the advice given to the students when developing their evidence-based portfolios. Students are asked to consider the:

- Relevance
- Appropriateness, and
- Learning which was demonstrated through each piece of evidence collected.

To assist with this they are then advised to examine the evidence in relation to the following criteria:

- Authenticity – does the evidence indicate clearly that the practitioner knows what hc/shc claims to know?
- Validity – does the evidence relate directly to the learning outcome?
- Directness – is the focus sharp and clear?
- Breadth – does the evidence relate to wider considerations?
- Currency – does the evidence demonstrate that the practitioner is up to date with contemporary developments and research?
- Sufficiency – is the evidence sufficient to demonstrate that learning outcomes have been met?
- Quality – is the standard of work equivalent to the level of the work? *Quantity* does not necessarily equate with *quality*.

In a further attempt to maintain focus and direction, students are advised to collect the evidence in stages:

Stage 1 – involves the selection of two case studies/episodes of care
Stage 2 – involves, where possible, gathering the evidence around the two selected case studies/episodes of care
Stage 3 – involves clearly stating why and how the evidence presented relates to the competency. The *connection* between the evidence and the competency must be explicit. A variety of evidence is acceptable providing the above criteria are met, and may include:

- Literature reviews
- Lesson plans
- Care plans
- Letters/referral forms

- Reflective accounts and analysis of these
- Critical incidents and analysis of these
- Tape recorded discussions
- Diary entries.

The evidence presented may be from either a macro or micro perspective. Types of data may include:

- Qualitative
- Quantitative
- Demographic
- Epidemiological
- Experiential.

The guidelines clearly state that evidence *isn't*:

- Full copies of assignments
- Photocopies of journal articles/book chapters
- Patient information leaflets
- Trust publications

(unless the student was originally involved in development or publication).

Comment

At present, portfolios at the University of Northumbria at Newcastle are assessed on a pass/fail basis. This is a collaborative process which involves the student, the mentor and the university teacher meeting in practice to explore clinical competencies and the evidence provided to support these. Central to the process is the mentor's role in observing clinical competence in practice. These tripartite meetings (of which there are a minimum of five over the duration of the course) are used to encourage reflection on practice and critical dialogue over what constitutes evidence and best practice. This process of evidence collection is further developed through the Higher Award initiative (see Chapter 7.)

Although students often express initial apprehension with portfolio development, this soon passes when they realise that they will be supported through the process. Many have stated that the process has helped them to think more critically about what they are doing and the rationale underpinning their actions. Through engaging in this process we are hopefully facilitating the development of reflective practitioners who will be able to begin to articulate some of that knowledge underpinning and embedded in practice. However, at present we have only anecdotal evidence to support this.

Summary

However practice is assessed, there can be no question that within programmes leading to a specialist practice award, the assessment of practice makes a clear statement about competencies in action. To over-assess or under-assess does no favours to the student, the public or employers.

The mentor is faced with an infinite list of assessable variables on a daily basis, provides immediate feedback and suggests innovative, developmental remedies. Assessment decisions made by the mentor are fundamental to the future of quality patient and client care; to make the right decision requires an extensive repertoire of assessment skills and a large degree of flexibility.

Part 3
Practice: Opportunities and Challenges

This final part of the book focuses on the reality of practice in specialist community practice. We have felt it important to begin by presenting a double chapter that discusses issues of relevance to all practitioners and mentors, whoever they are, wherever they are and whatever the practice – evidence-based practice and research-minded practice. Whereas we have all probably accepted that evidence-based practice is a must, we strangely seem to have adopted a less enthusiastic approach to the research which underpins most of the evidence base. Joanne Bennett takes us on a journey through the concepts of evidence, letting Chris Wibberley and Linda Dack present their vision of promoting research in practice.

After eight contributors have presented chapters that specify the issues facing particular specialist community practices, a specialist community practitioner graduate and a mentor provide us with an honest glimpse of 'what it's really like'. The penultimate chapter is up-to-date navigation of practice for those who want to tackle the 'wicked issues'.

While Chapters 10–17 focus on specific specialist practitioner roles, many of the issues that are raised within, for example, 'health visiting' are relevant to all students and all mentors. Thus we advise readers, rather than just selecting 'their' chapter, to consider what other disciplines have to say. Mentors, and other teachers, may learn much from ideas raised from outside practice.

Chapter 9

The Evidence and Research Base for Practice

In this two-part chapter, the issues that form the basis of practice are explored. First, Joanne Bennett provides the background to evidence-based practice and identifies what is meant by 'evidence'. Although there may be justification for utilising that rather intangible 'professional experience' as part of the evidence base, it remains weak, subjective and disputed evidence until backed up by systematic study. Chris Wibberley and Linda Dack move in here to explore how practitioners can be research involved and how they can encourage their practices to develop a research culture. Chris Wibberley has a wealth of experience within HEI research development, evaluating research and supporting practitioner-researchers. Linda Dack has been involved in developing research-mindedness and a research culture in practice settings.

PART 1   EVIDENCE-BASED PRACTICE
Joanne Bennett

Introduction

The broad concept of evidence-based practice has become a common topic of discussion in nursing, and its roots can be traced back to evidence-based medicine (Reynolds 2000). However, confusion often arises about what is meant by evidence-based practice. This section will address this through briefly exploring the development of evidence-based practice in general, before moving on to clarify what constitutes the evidence-base in nursing. For those needing to explore these issues further, Trinder and Reynolds (2000) provide a comprehensive and critical collection of work in this area.

The development of evidence-based practice

Reynolds (2000) describes how the gap between research and practice in medicine has had a tendency to be uneasy with the translation of research findings into practice, being erratic and unsystematic. She suggests that proponents of this approach claim that evidence-based medicine developed to bridge that gap and she goes on to highlight how.

First, evidence-based practice distinguishes between research which is of direct significance to practice, and that which is not. Second, it provides a structured set of rules for evaluating research and its appropriateness, or otherwise, to clinical practice. Third, it provides a framework for making decisions based on the best evidence. In doing so, it emphasises professional responsibility, the need for decision-making to be explicit and transparent, the changing hierarchical and incomplete nature of evidence and the importance of critical appraisal skills (Reynolds 2000).

Evidence-based nursing

Developments in evidence-based nursing have mirrored those in evidence-based medicine in a number of ways. First, evidence-based nursing grew out of recognition that despite the recommendations made in the Briggs Report (DHSS 1977) which called for nursing to become a research-based profession, there was little evidence to suggest that this was happening. Second, Blomfield and Hardy (2000) point out the similarities in the definitions of evidence-based nursing to those of evidence-based medicine, comparing that of DiCenso *et al.* (1998) with that of Sackett *et al.* (1997). For example, they quote DiCenso *et al.* (1998, p.119) who define evidence-based nursing as:

'The process by which nurses make clinical decisions using the best available research evidence, their clinical expertise and patient preferences, in the context of available resources.'

This is almost identical to Sackett *et al.* (1997, p.71) who state that evidence-based medicine is:

'The conscientious, explicit and judicious use of current best evidence in making decisions about the care of individual patients, based on skills which allow the doctor to evaluate both personal experience and external evidence in a systematic and objective manner.'

Third, the process in both nursing and medicine involves generating evidence, followed by the critical appraisal of the evidence and dissemination (Blomfield & Hardy 2000).

What constitutes evidence?

At a glance the argument so far seems fairly straightforward. It is when attempts are made to describe the evidence-base of nursing that difficulties are encountered. Despite the definitions offered above, which suggest that clinical expertise and patient preferences are central to the process, the overriding message from our medical colleagues is that quantitative research, often in the form of randomised control trials, provides a stronger evidence-base than qualitative and interpretative research. The interpretation of what constitutes the evidence-base in nursing, and arguably medicine too, needs to be much broader than this to address the complexity and artistry of practice.
It is at this point that we need to visit the debate presented in Chapter 5,

where the knowledge base of nursing is discussed and strategies explored to begin to uncover and articulate knowledge embedded in practice. It is only when we reach this point that we will truly begin to combine consumer preferences with other forms of knowledge. This warrants a move away from exploring the evidence-base through the over-reliance on the more traditional methods of quantitative research to the integration of interpretive methods that attempt to capture the complexity of practice. One possible route to this is the development of a research culture which encourages diversity and embraces a willingness to think and work in different ways.

Part 2 RESEARCH-MINDED PRACTICE AND RESEARCH CULTURE
Dr Christopher Wibberley and Linda Dack

Introduction

Although research is linked to evidence-based practice, the concept of research-minded practice may be more difficult to grasp for those practitioners who are not currently involved in research activity. Our argument is that unless a clear research culture exists, evidence-based practice may not occur, or may be thought to occur but in effect be handled inappropriately or inaccurately. Additionally, it is common practice within nursing and health visiting for practitioners to rely on others to carry out research relevant to practice. But, as practitioner roles are constantly developing and increasing personal and professional accountability, a continued reliance on others to provide evidence and the research base with which to develop practice does not seem to be a sound state of affairs. As part of the mentor's role is developing practice (UKCC 2000a), involvement in research focused on practice, however small (for example, user satisfaction with extant services), must be considered to be part of the role. The 'research' role should not be viewed as an extra burden but another 'skill' of lead practitioners.

The question for nursing and health visiting is how can it encourage its practitioners to embrace the principle that research is an intrinsic part of their working life and indispensable for good practice? In other words, how can a research culture be fostered and furthermore can the existence of such a culture be explicitly demonstrated and so monitored? In this part of the chapter we explore what we mean by research and the form that research-minded practice is likely to take for the majority of practitioners. First we must point out that the following account is based on our experiences of developing research-mindedness and a research culture in practice; hence there is a lack of reference to theory.

The meaning of research for those in practice

The question for practitioners (and academics) is how to characterise research that is focused on practice. It is our view that the following three key points act as appropriate descriptors of such research:

- Practice-based research can be considered to be a process of disciplined enquiry, involving the collection and analysis of data relating to an identified practice-related issue.
- The intended outcome of research is relevant description, explanation, generalisation or prediction which contributes to the study of either practice itself and/or of interventions which are a part of this practice.
- The research will contribute to practice in terms of theory, the application of theory and/or the application of skills within that field of practice.

For the mentor the emphasis should be in relation to critical appraisal or application of research in relation to the identified needs of practice. Furthermore, the primary consideration of the mentor, in terms of those for whom they are educationally responsible, is in ensuring that their practice is demonstrably grounded in evidence, thus providing a good example to the novice specialist practitioner. In providing such an example, though, it is also vital that mentors make clear the role of clinical experience and expertise in developing and applying the evidence base; it is the ability to undertake such mediation that separates the mentor from their informed student. Thus, the mentor can be seen to engage with the evidence-base as opposed to merely being aware of it.

In some cases an individual practitioner may begin by questioning an aspect of their own practice, may attempt to review the evidence upon which their actions are based and may undertake some small-scale research if the evidence is found wanting. For example, a district nurse finds there is no local strategy for elder abuse and subsequently carries out a small-scale study of strategies available within the National Health Service Management Executive (NHSME) region. This leads to the development of a local policy based on best available practice. The practice of the district nurse and colleagues is then influenced by the findings of the review or small-scale research.

However, if the situation warrants, the practitioner may develop a proposal for more substantial research or systematic review (for example a study of the prevention of pressure sores within community settings), and will seek collaboration and/or funding to carry it out. This will require more formal involvement at a local level and/or possibly at a regional or national level. Some practitioners may also become involved as either experts or representatives of their specialism in formal processes within the NHS research and development funding initiative.

All the levels of involvement noted above demonstrate research-minded practice in some form.

Research-minded practice

To maintain research-minded practice in a given group of practitioners whatever the organisational structure, the grouping needs to contain or have access to one or more people to provide 'research leadership'. Groupings of practitioners may be based on professional background or specialism, client groups, service delivery or some other factor. 'Research leadership' may be provided from outside the grouping, but common sense and our own experience in the practice setting would suggest that they need to be accessible and credible to those who are research engaged. Research leads should be involved in other research networks, and should have contact with other research leads from within and/or outside their own organisations. Research engaged staff should be very much a part of the grouping they are attached to on a day-to-day basis, although they may also be involved with research engaged staff in other research networks.

Personnel are a key element in fostering a culture within which research is valued and research-minded practice considered the norm. In the next section we will look at other factors which can be considered to help foster a research culture and at ways in which mentors can assess/monitor the existence of such a culture. Given that mentors should be encouraging those for whom they are educationally responsible to be research-minded, it is important that they have some means of assessing that they are themselves operating within an environment that fosters a research culture.

Fostering a research culture

A research culture can be considered to exist when the environment within which people operate leads them to accept the research process as a valid, valued and, in fact, integral part of their professional practice and that of others with whom they work. Thus, one would expect to find a visible research community, access to research training and on-going advice and support, and availability of appropriate resources – facilities and equipment.

A visible research community may be demonstrated, amongst other things, by:

- Identification of groupings of staff with associated research leads, research engaged and research aware staff
- Involvement of staff in research interest groups within and across practitioner groups which may be organised from both inside and outside the practitioner's own organisation
- Identification of how the activity of groupings of staff fits within an overall research plan for the organisation(s) to which the staff belong
- Staff publications in professional and academic journals, relating to research they have been involved in or the application of research within the practice setting
- A record of bids for funding to external bodies for research activity

- Involvement in local, national and international conferences as both speakers/workshop leaders and participants.

Access to research training and on-going advice and support should include, amongst other things:

- A training needs assessment which clearly identifies research needs of staff
- Regular programmes including research training and research updates, which are well-received by staff
- Clear routes of access to specialist research advice and support, including named responsible staff within and, where appropriate, outside the organisation.

Availability of appropriate resources, facilities and equipment should include access to:

- Library, internet and computing resources
- Audio-visual recording equipment
- Appropriate software for data analysis
- Quiet rooms where interviews can be carried out/interest groups can be held
- Time allocated to research activity, with an indication of the proportion of their role that this should relate to.

Monitoring the above (or similar) factors in itself can be seen as demonstrating commitment by an organisation to take research seriously – and so should be encouraged.

Conclusion

In writing this part of the chapter, we have been aware of the irony that there is a paucity of research into research-minded practice. However, we have attempted to outline some principles that we hope will help the reader come to grips with what research-minded practice means for those working in and around the health and social care sector.

Chapter 10
General Practice Nursing

Sarah Mattocks

Educational preparation for the specialist community practitioner in general practice nursing is developing rapidly and there is considerable interest in the mentor role. Sarah Mattocks has inside experience of the issues that will and may affect mentors working within a profession that enjoys a unique employment structure and practice culture. Through her experience Sarah is able to present strategies for managing learning in practice for general practice nursing students.

Introduction

The history and culture of general medical practice, the role of the practice nurse, the status of the specialist practitioner qualification, and the nature of current and developing health service structures and boundaries are among the factors contributing to the complex environment within which mentorship in practice nursing has to be negotiated. For this reason I will start by raising some of the key contextual issues, before moving on to discuss the management and evaluation of mentoring and to illustrate the challenges and opportunities these present for the mentor.

General medical practice and the role of the practice nurse

In undertaking the mentor role in practice nursing it is important to have an understanding of the history and culture of general practice and the evolution of the discipline. For those needing to explore this further, Damant *et al.* (1994) and Edwards (1999) provide helpful background reading. Issues of particular relevance include the influence of employment and management structures on the provision of education and training for nurses in general practice, and expectations and scope of the practice nurse role as this continues to evolve (ENB 1995; Poulton 1997; Lunt & Atkin 1999).

Perspectives on education and training needs for nurses working in general practice vary, particularly in relation to undertaking the specialist practitioner award for general practice nurses (UKCC 1998). The main reason for this is that the specialist practitioner award is non-mandatory for nurses employed in general practice. The diversity of expectations and role development is evident if we explore at one end of the spectrum GPs' perspectives; GPs may be more concerned with immediate operational issues from a medical perspective, for example the delivery of specialist clinical services such as chronic disease management. At the other end, Health Authority sponsors may be more concerned with the strategic direction of nursing and with the acquisition of clinical leadership and practice development competencies, preparing nurses to shape the future of health care delivery in primary care (DoH 1999a). Similarly views expressed by practice nurses are varied, reflecting the considerable diversity in the practice nurse population in terms of experience, career development and vision for the future of the discipline and their own professional role.

In many instances GPs (and non-nursing managers) have acted as gatekeepers to professional training and education for the practice nurses they employ. It may be argued that the GP both as employer (in most cases) and in terms of the relationship between medicine and nursing, still enjoys the greatest influence in the decision-making process at practice level. With the introduction of Primary Care Groups (PCGs) and Primary Care Trusts (PCTs) (DoH 1997a) and the re-examination of professional roles in both medicine and nursing (DoH 1999a), the climate is set to change. However, for some practice nurses their professional role development may be a sensitive issue within the primary health care team (Edwards 1999). The non-mandatory status of the qualification adds to the potential hurdles for nurses arguing to undertake the award.

There are additional challenges for those wishing to undertake the course in terms of feasibility, in particular funding and replacement cover (where the nurse is already in post) and the provision for the practice component of the course. Even with more recent non-medical education and training (NMET) (DoH 1998b), money being dedicated through workforce development confederations for general practice nursing staff replacement costs – in reality finding an equivalent replacement to cover an existing practice nurse's study leave – remains difficult. In my experience many practice nurses find themselves making significant sacrifices to secure the support of their GP employer in undertaking the course. Examples include those already on part-time contracts agreeing to take on their own locum cover around course commitments, or using their day off for attendance at university.

The role of the mentor in practice nursing requires a high level of collaborative working in a rapidly changing and complex environment. An understanding of the context of general practice, development of the role of the practice nurse, and management of education and training will help better equip mentors to manage relationships sensitively and positively. I would argue that augmenting the role of a practice nurse to specialist practice (UKCC 1998) is in itself part of the overall change process, as is the continued evolution of infrastructures and processes to facilitate mentoring for this group, and it needs to be understood in this light.

Facilitating practice learning in general practice nursing

Models for implementation

A key factor in identifying an appropriate model for the implementation of mentorship is the recruitment and selection strategy adopted by Health Authorities and PCGs, together with the profile of the students seeking to undertake the course. Variations exist across the UK and depend on many and complex variables including the level of commitment demonstrated and innovation achieved by key stakeholders in creating the conditions necessary to promote mentorship and role development in practice nursing.

A learning contract negotiated with each student at the outset should identify key areas for development in specialist practice (UKCC 1998, pp.1–2, 13), together with the scope and level of autonomy to be achieved and how this can be facilitated. For students with prior experience and deemed competent within their current practice nursing role, there may be less need for direct supervision of care delivery and a greater emphasis on reflection and critical analysis. Conversely, for students who are relatively new to the environment of general practice, with little or no previous experience in general practice nursing, there will need to be greater input in terms of the acquisition of skills and knowledge in direct clinical care delivery, as well as on reflection and critical analysis.

The GPN students with whom I have worked in relation to the specialist practitioner award have all had experience in the role of practice nurse and arrangements to support them have taken account of this. Different practices (or trusts), usually employ mentors and their respective students, and a major challenge is presented by the practicalities involved in getting both in the same place at the same time to engage in the educational process. It may be wise, given the cross-boundary and inter-disciplinary nature of support for practice nurses undertaking the course, to clarify and make explicit the responsibilities and lines of reporting and accountability at the outset. Issues of confidentiality and anonymity need to be addressed and it is important to clarify on what basis and with whom information about the student's performance should be shared.

The students have undertaken the practice component on a part-time basis in their own area of practice with their employing GP. Advantages of this model include the opportunity to profile the needs of the practice population in the context of local Health Improvement Programmes (HImPs) and to target specific areas of role development to meet patient needs. This also affords the opportunity to engage practice colleagues in the process of nursing role development in the context of the wider team. Disadvantages, however, include the problems associated with role ambiguity for the nurse within the practice (Handy 1993). Designated time for the development of new aspects of specialist practice and the role transition to specialist practitioner may be difficult to protect when working in their 'home' practice. Case study 10.1 illustrates the arrangements negotiated and put in place.

Kate had been a practice nurse for eight years when she started the course, and had developed her knowledge of the GPN role through experiential learning and formal study at diploma level. The nurse advisor from the sponsoring authority undertook a facilitation role in negotiating with the GP employer regarding the commitment required from the practice. In liaison with the course leader the nurse advisor secured the support of an appropriate practitioner from another general practice who was willing and able to take on the role of mentor in an independent capacity, making arrangements for remuneration through locally agreed mechanisms. The mentor, Charlotte, had herself undertaken the specialist practitioner course and was well placed to guide and direct Kate through the learning process.

Given Kate's prior experiential and accredited learning the implementation of the practice component was based on that of clinical supervision (see Chapter 6), with negotiated activities for taught and observed practice including reciprocal arrangements to base these in their respective practices, within the constraints imposed by professional indemnity. In liaison with Kate's GP employer, given the diversity of practice nurse training needs, Charlotte was able to draw upon her professional networks to complement her own skills and expertise, providing mentoring and experience to enable Kate to achieve her negotiated clinical and professional learning needs.

Case study 10.1 Arranging appropriate mentorship and placement

The process of learning, teaching and assessment and the role of the mentor

In terms of the learning, teaching and assessment process it is important to develop a good rapport and relationship of trust between the mentor and student, and time taken to develop this is an important investment. This creates the conditions necessary for the student to respond positively to being challenged, and to be able to examine and evaluate their practice in a climate of support and safety. At the same time it is important to be clear about roles and responsibilities within the relationship, particularly with regard to the assessment of practice (see Chapter 8).

The concern sometimes expressed regarding what to 'teach' an experienced practice nurse, particularly in relation to specialist practice, can be explored within tripartite discussions with the university teacher. However, in my experience it has been useful to approach this in terms of encouraging these practitioners to uncover and articulate the nursing knowledge that informs their current practice (see Chapter 5), and bring forward the evidence to support this. This is invariably a challenging developmental process, demanding energy and perseverance both from the student and the mentor.

The following scenario captures key features of the educational process in action. Here the mentor helps shape the practice setting and harnesses her own expertise to provide a positive learning environment in which the student can gain the knowledge, experience and skills in clinical care and gain confidence in leadership and practice development.

Laura had been in post as a practice nurse for two years when she started the course and already provided a clinic service for people with diabetes together with other members of the team. However, this aspect of her practice was one which both Laura and Susan (the mentor) agreed could be further developed to respond to patient needs. Findings of an audit of diabetic care undertaken by Laura highlighted areas of concern, with a number of patients showing poor diabetic control as well as infrequent and erratic attendance for specialist clinical care. Laura's reaction to this was, among other things, one of anxiety in relation to quality and standards and a sense of professional vulnerability and wavering confidence in her specialist clinical practice and practice nurse role.

Key tasks for Susan were to encourage and support Laura both through the reflective process and in developing her critical thinking skills. This involved firstly analysing the specific health needs of this client group. Susan encouraged Laura to gather and analyse data from a variety of sources to identify a gap in the service. This process included the analysis of selected critical incidents (see Chapter 5). It became clear that it was patients with mental health problems who were documented as receiving the least care and having the worst diabetic control. An action plan was then devised that included Laura initiating collaborative links with the community psychiatric nurses in the area, and taking a lead in practice development across organisational and professional boundaries. With the support of her university teacher, an enquiry-based approach (see Chapter 9) was adopted. This enabled Laura to learn more about mental health problems and how these might affect attendance for diabetic care and the ability to respond to advice and treatment, and to consider the principles of effective collaboration and how this could be promoted in the health care team. This knowledge enabled her to tailor the service more effectively to address the specific needs of this client group. Debates in this area were also developed in the classroom. Susan was able to evaluate Laura's performance on a *continuous basis*, through observation of clinical practice, critical discussion and analysis, and reviewing the evidence presented by Laura in her portfolio (see Chapter 8 for more detail on practice learning portfolios).

Case study 10.2 Facilitating development for an experienced practitioner

Evaluating mentorship in general practice nursing

The structure and process of mentorship for practice nurses undertaking this professional award is constantly evolving and needs continuing evaluation and review. Discussion and debate around models for implementing mentoring are essential, in terms of strengths, limitations and strategies for the future. The challenge of facilitating the development of nurses new to general practice is a particular concern. The diversity and level of autonomy that can be achieved within specialist practice will be influenced by the appropriateness of the model for implementing mentorship, as well as by the duration of the course. It is important to establish realistic expectations and the concept of life-long learning together, with the value of transferable skills (ENB 1995) explored with students and employers.

In my experience, with established practice nurses and their mentors, the key issues raised have tended to focus on logistic factors and the extent to which arrangements agreed in principle, for example for protected time, are respected. The scope and flexibility needed to gain further skills and therapeutic techniques in specialist practice are only as good as the local infrastructures to secure this. Erosion of this would present even greater concern should the student be new to the discipline. The way in which the needs of practice nurses are reflected in terms of curriculum design and delivery within the theoretical element of the course is likewise an area of continuing evaluation.

Both mentors and students particularly highlight the difficulty in arranging mutually convenient times to spend together for the practice period, and the way that nursing services in general practice are usually arranged can make this particularly difficult, where clinics are booked well in advance. Forward planning for the necessary protected time and developmental activities is needed. Travelling time between practices (geographical proximity therefore being a factor) also has to be built in, an available room for private discussion secured, and a strategy to avoid inappropriate interruptions agreed within the practice. These factors mean that success in terms of the practical structuring of the arrangements has so far rested heavily on the commitment, flexibility and goodwill shown by mentors towards their students. Many, for example, offer telephone contact and discussion between sessions.

For mentors in practice nursing there are further hurdles to negotiate. Access to formal courses of preparation for the role can be difficult to achieve for a number of reasons including, again, being released from practice commitments to engage in professional development activities. This issue requires urgent consideration, particularly given the new standards for the preparation of teachers of nursing, midwifery and health visiting (UKCC 2000a). Likewise, mentor meetings convened at the university can be extremely difficult to schedule into an already busy workload, meaning peer support and review need to be achieved through other means. Here the role of the personal tutor is important in being flexible and available to discuss specific issues as these arise. Mentors also need to consider how best to develop their own networks of support. Multiple sites again being an issue, it is sometimes easier and just as valuable to meet up with mentors supporting community students from other disciplines where they are based in the same practice.

In evaluating the educational process a number of themes emerge. One is the importance of good rapport between the mentor and student. In my experience students need a great deal of emotional support in terms of role transition to specialist practice. This is most noticeable in terms of breaking out of the professional isolation so often felt by practice nurses within the primary health care team, developing collaborative links, becoming more assertive, developing leadership skills, and managing practice development. Here it is the personal qualities of the mentor that are often most valued. Another theme is that both mentors and their students tend to show greater confidence in managing the process where the mentors themselves have undertaken a similar course of preparation at degree level. Finally, students value the mentor as a role model of the reflective practitioner, critical thinker, and life-long learner. From the mentors' points of view participation in the preparation of these students and the educational process, whilst demanding, is valuable in terms of their own professional development.

Conclusion

It is to be hoped that changes in the structure of the health service and increasing influence of specialist practitioners in primary health care will help contribute to shifts in the learning culture of general practice. This in turn should promote greater flexibility in implementing and delivering appropriate practice education for practice nursing in future.

The investment made by mentors in this new discipline within specialist practice is high, and the return to students is clear. Mary, an experienced practice nurse, reflecting on the skill of her mentor in facilitating her development, commented:

'I was beginning to reappraise the overall context of my professional environment. I was developing an open mind and therefore able to appreciate the broader picture of how self, colleagues and organisation were integrated ... I knew my former self-perception was fading, that of passive practice nurse, and the transition towards specialist practitioner was occurring'.

Reflecting on completion of the course Mary commented, 'I really didn't think the course would change me – but it did!'. For mentors, enabling students to fulfill their potential as specialist practitioners in general practice nursing equally brings rewards, professionally, personally and, most importantly, for patients in primary health care.

Chapter 11

Community Mental Health Nursing

Maureen Deacon

Recently community mental health nursing has managed a great deal of change and doubtless will continue to do so. Within this educational field the mentor may meet a variety of students from a wide range of different community mental health practices. In this chapter Maureen Deacon has managed to combine an informal study of students and mentors, and integrates a critical evaluation of theory with the reality of practice.

Introduction

The aim of this chapter is to examine critically the factors that enable mentors of community mental health nurses (CMHNs) to carry out this particular role successfully. This role is, of course, contextualised by the broader roles that mentors play as practitioners, managers, leaders and colleagues in increasingly complex multi-disciplinary and multi-agency mental health teams. It is also framed by the rather ambiguous status of the specialist practitioner award in community mental health nursing; this, I will argue, adds to the challenge of the work.

My starting position is that it is hard to do the job of mentor well. It demands commitment, enthusiasm, generosity and stamina. It is often invisible work, taken for granted, which in many organisations you will be expected to 'absorb' into your already busy schedule. This, however, will be a familiar state of affairs which you may already be well experienced in managing. The good news is that the work can be incredibly rewarding and play an important part in your continuing professional development. As a mentor recently put it: 'It keeps me on my toes – it means that I have to keep up to date and it gives me access to all sorts of material that I wouldn't see and think about otherwise'.

Two groups of people have helpfully shared with me their experiences of mentoring, in preparation for writing this chapter; a current group of mentors completed a survey based around the question, 'What do you need to do the job well?' and a group of established CMHN students joined me in a discussion concerning what *they* needed from their mentors. In this way I hope to reflect the perspectives of the different stakeholders in this process. To set these personal experiences in context, I will initially examine the ambiguous status of the CMHN award and the practical consequences of this ambiguity.

The specialist practitioner award and community mental health nursing

Educational preparation for CMHNs has an interesting history which has been carefully analysed by White (1990). Using a documentary method of analysis, White (1990, p.289) sets out a chronological account of this history and powerfully makes the case that CMHN education:

'... has been characterized by a series of difficult and essentially unsuccessful struggles to secure and protect adequate finance for an effective system of post-registration education.'

This lack of funding is reflexively bound up with the non-mandatory nature of the qualification. The fact that a registered mental nurse can be employed as a CMHN without the qualification (at any grade between E and H in my experience) works against the likelihood of such funding being prioritised. Bowers (1996) and Hannigan (1999) provide thought-provoking examination of the trends in recruitment to CMHN courses, the latter author noting 'tentative evidence' that there is a decline in recruitment nationally. They also raise important questions concerning the variation of course content, observing that different centres of education offer a diverse range of study topics as well as shared issues. Just as White (1990) did before them, they paint a picture of CMHN education as an entity, which is vulnerable on a number of fronts. These include the practical difficulties of moving the course to degree level when many CMHNs are not currently at diploma level, and the absence of nationally agreed detailed curriculum content. The latter of these is compounded by the ongoing debate concerning the 'proper' role of CMHNs.

There are two threads from this earlier work that I intend to examine further in terms of their practical consequences for mentors. These concern the non-mandatory status of the specialist community practitioner qualification and the dispute concerning the work of CMHNs.

The non-mandatory status of the qualification is rapidly identifiable in the classroom. Nurses become CMHN students from a wide variety of employment positions. G grade students who have been in the job for years sit next to an E grade who has previously worked on an acute admission ward; an 'H' grade team leader of a specialist dementia service shares a desk with an 'E' grade working in a primary mental health care team. Behind them sits a forensic specialist who divides his time between a court diversion scheme and care co-ordinating a highly risky group of people who are subject to restriction orders under The Mental Health Act 1983. This diversity of students, who are examples from my recent teaching experience, indicates that neatly identifying just who CMHNs are, is problematic (Bowers 1997). This mix provides tremendous opportunity for shared learning in the university setting but provides a particular set of challenges for the mentor. Just as there is no 'standard' CMHN there can be no standard mentoring package put together and delivered 'off the shelf'.

Clearly, helping the students to identify their own professional learning needs is the place to begin. Engaging in this process and then moving it on from identifying general development needs to the practicalities of making it happen, is strenuous work. Essentially this process demands the skills of clinical supervision within the context of an authoritative, accountable process.

Barry began the course 20 years into his nursing career, having spent the last seven as a G grade CMHN in a community mental health team. Sarah, his mentor, had been his colleague for five years. Barry was keen to learn but found it hard to move away from the 'I've been there and got the scars to prove it' position (Kadushin 1968). Sarah felt frustrated with Barry but was reluctant to challenge him; in terms of years served, he was actually more experienced than her and she had a lot of respect for his skills. Furthermore, she could see how anxious he was beginning to get about the academic work involved in the course and this added to her fears of pushing him. However, Sarah was aware that there was little point in Barry doing the course if he was going to be practising in exactly the same way at the end of it.

The way forward was to change the unspoken rules of their professional relationship. Sarah sought supervision with this dilemma and worked out a creative strategy. She asked Barry to come and observe her doing a new assessment and to give her constructive criticism on her performance. From this she wanted them to negotiate a structured method for critically examining practice. Together they came up with five questions that could form the basis of all their casework discussion:

- What did you do?
- Why did you do it that way?
- What went well?
- What did you struggle with?
- What will you do differently next time?

All these questions were designed to connect theory and practice, or as Holloway (1995) more eloquently describes the process: 'adapting the known methods'. This strategy (which Heron (1990) would probably call a 'catalytic' intervention, while Papp (1983) would use the notion of 'reframing') did not entirely resolve Sarah's discomfort at playing the role of 'judge' with a colleague but it did enable her to make accountable judgements about Barry's progress. Barry, on the other hand, relished the challenge and appreciated the opportunity to examine his practice in relation to its evidence base.

Case study 11.1 Mentorship for an experienced practitioner

A further ramification of the non-mandatory status of the qualification is the concomitant level of esteem with which the course may be held locally. Fundamentally this boils down to the attitude of 'why bother?'. Whilst it may be possible for the mentor and the student to resist its negative implications, it can be wearing on the spirit, especially when the going gets tough. The best strategy is preventative. Given that most helping professionals are 'tuned into' a working conceptual environment of caring (Deacon 1998), the mentor can explicitly ask for the team's help in supporting the student before the placement begins. This is especially important when the placement is in the student's usual working environment, where they need to make on-going negotiated transitions between organisationally incongruent roles. Discussing the practicalities of how they can help by working through some of the issues that might arise will give the mentor a strong platform for resolving any future difficulties.

The role of the community mental health nurse

The debate concerning the *proper* role of the CMHN is indisputably important and one that a student cannot avoid engaging with during their education. Some high moral ground has been captured during the documented 'care wars' (Tilley 1997, p.203) but practitioners have to find their way through what Schön (1990) refers to as the 'swampy lowlands' of practice. This poses a difficult dilemma for some mentors: should they facilitate the student's development in relation to their current and future role in the organisation, or should they orientate their development towards a more abstract but officially approved role? One pedagogic solution to this quandary has been to teach *principles* of CMHN practice but the mentor has to work it through in the context of their and their student's organisational reality. For example, it is deemed 'correct' in the current climate for CMHNs to develop their skills in family interventions concerning a family member with schizophrenia. Given the complexity of these skills and their evidence base a CMHN student could easily spend a large chunk of their placement time concentrating on this area. However, it may be the case that the student is doing their placement in a primary mental health care team, where a diverse range of mental health problems will be encountered. Skills required in this setting will share some fundamentally important ground with those in family interventions, including for example: engaging people in the therapeutic process; doing careful bio-psychosocial assessments which lead to an appropriate and effective care plan; and co-working in a complex organisational environment and employing effective recording processes. However, there will also be different skills required and students will have different needs.

(In the north-west of England, services seem to be organising their work with people between the ages of 16 and 65 around the categories of 'severe and enduring mental health problems' and 'primary care'. In practice this seems to mean one service for people with psychotic disorders and one for everybody else (the nature of 'everybody' being determined by locally constructed criteria).)

Julie, an experienced CMHN, wanted to develop her skills in working with people who frequently engaged in deliberate self-harm. She had observed that this was a poorly served and unpopular client group who often caused mayhem in her service. Julie's mentor discussed this with the university teacher during a placement visit. The tutor suggested that Julie investigate Linehan *et al.*'s (1991) dialectical behaviour therapy model for people with borderline personality disorder as a 'starting point'. Julie subsequently followed this 'thread' through a number of her course modules and achieved her learning objectives.

Case study 11.2 Creative mentorship

There really is no definitive, prescriptive answer to the dilemma of precisely what each individual CMHN student should systematically investigate beyond broad, evidence-based principles of skilled practice. My view is that CMHNs should develop their practice in a way that relates to their own world of work and the future development of that organisation. They need to develop skills that will benefit their client group. As Price (1999) has observed, the development of individual skills is only worthwhile if the organisational infrastructure allows those skills to be used effectively.

Having examined the ambiguous context of CMHN education I will now turn to the perspectives of mentors and their students on the question of what helps the role to develop successfully.

What helps mentors carry out the role successfully?

The mentor view

Mentors were asked to consider the resources that they required within the structured categories of their organisational context, their individual professional characteristics and the educational institution.

Organisationally two main themes emerged. The first theme concerned their relationship with their manager: there is a need to have the role valued and recognised in terms of workload and, at times, the mentor may need to be assertive in order to protect the student from inappropriate organisational demands. Mentors want to have a choice about whether or not they take on the role and feel that there should be a measure of reciprocity in terms of the organisation supporting *their* development.

The second theme concerned the need for a supportive environment. This meant colleagues taking an interest and having a good understanding of the course (one participant referred to this eloquently as colleagues having been 'academically socialised'). It meant working in a team where multi-disciplinary colleagues were willing to provide learning opportunities; and having access to good quality clinical supervision and the opportunity to meet up with other local mentors.

With reference to the required individual professional characteristics, what emerged resonated strongly with the literature concerning the qualities of good clinical supervisors. These included: 'Able to inspire, encourage, motivate and reassure', 'Confidence and experience in the specialist community practitioner role', and 'Able to cope with challenge confidently'. These qualities are often taken for granted in practice and can be challenging to maintain consistently throughout a lengthy placement. Faugier (1992) emphasises the importance of trust in an effective supervisory relationship. This notion of trust is seen to be the bedrock of effective mentoring – the student needs to have faith in the integrity of their mentor's professional skills and their personal qualities.

Resources required from the educational institution analytically fell into two categories: course organisation and personal contact. Mentors need timely information about the course and clear expectations of their role, regular contact through study days, placement visits and support meetings. Personally they call for accessible help and prompt action when problems arise, the opportunity to consider their own educational needs and acknowledgement that the role is demanding. There are no great surprises here but this observation belies the complexities involved in having these needs met. Clearly, the 'soon to be' mentor would be well advised to closely consider these issues when preparing to take on the role. Let us now turn to the students' perspectives on what they need from their mentor.

The student view

The students' perspectives resonated with those expressed by the mentors in many ways. There is a 'parallel process' (Halgin 1986) evident between what mentors need and what their students need from them. Organisationally students wanted their mentors to have 'clout', that is, they wanted them to be in a position to protect the students from inappropriate demands and to help them gain access to learning experiences. The maintenance of clean organisational role boundaries was particularly important for part-time students. They suggested that practical strategies such as separating clinical supervision for their 'student' casework from their 'ordinary' casework were helpful.

In the context of their supervisory relationship they found it helpful if they shared experiences of degree level study. One student suggested: 'they know what is expected of us and they can understand what we're going through'. Importantly they expected the mentor to take the lead in 'sorting out the role if it had been previously different' (for example, if they had been colleagues beforehand) and expected that having sorted it out the mentor should remain consistent and be generous with their expert practitioner guidance. A 'three party' meeting was suggested between students, their mentors and the university teachers early on in the course so that these issues could be jointly examined.

The most strikingly different issue that the students raised was the need to be challenged by their mentors. They deeply appreciated the level of support that they were given but believed that in order to develop as practitioners they needed to be asked difficult and uncomfortable questions about the rationale for, and the evidence base of, their practice. Having the opportunity to account for their work was the key to their development. This echoes my own experience that mentors tend to be extremely enthusiastic about the skills of their students. This positive approach provides an excellent foundation for learning and is a secure base for constructive challenge. It seems to be deeply embedded in nursing culture that challenge is negative, unpleasant and personally destructive (if approached punitively it can be but we need to draw a clear line between healthy, respectful challenge and being 'told off'). Mentors should discuss this issue with their students and confidently negotiate a strategy that promotes a learning relationship that is comfortably safe and supportive and powerfully challenging. Bringing this off successfully not only contributes to this specific learning experience but is an essential component of promoting a good practice culture.

Conclusion

In critically examining the factors that enable mentors to carry out their role successfully two broad themes have been investigated: the status of the specialist community practitioner award in mental health nursing and the perspectives of a group of course 'consumers'. The latter will share much in common with other categories of community nurses. The essential skills of providing high quality learning environments and learning relationships cut across professional role demarcations. It is the practical accomplishment of situating those skills into an organisational and professional context in a way that enables an individual student to develop, that is 'the difference that makes a difference'. This will have to be uniquely accomplished on each and every occasion that the mentor and their student jointly produce their learning environment. This will remain the case no matter how structured or unstructured the assessment materials provided by the educational institution, no matter what the dominant nursing discourse concerning the proper role of the CMHN suggests and no matter just how ambiguous the status of the award is within the profession.

To summarise, being a successful mentor is a difficult but rewarding role that requires the same skills as your average supernurse! These skills may be largely taken for granted and organisationally invisible. We should not allow this to trivialise or undermine the importance of the role. People with mental health problems deserve the best possible care that we can deliver and that work requires high quality life-long learners.

Chapter 12

Community Learning Disability Nursing

Peggy Cooke

Peggy Cooke has been involved with the education of community learning disability nursing students for many years. This chapter focuses on the need for 'would be' specialist practitioner students and mentors to gain support to undertake appropriate preparation. Throughout the chapter it is clear that organisational issues are paramount and some pragmatic strategies for managing seemingly impossible situations are provided.

Introduction

The role of the mentor in the support and assessment of community learning disability nursing students is still developing. In contrast to health visitors and district nurses, mentoring in community learning disability nursing is in its infancy. As Jukes (1994a) highlighted, 'there is no mandatory requirement for a community nurse in disability nursing to have a qualification for practice'. Without a requirement from the ENB for community learning disability nurses to have a community qualification or for students to be supported by a qualified practitioner, there has been no incentive for managers to allow practitioners to be prepared for the mentor role. This problem has been compounded by the lack of a clearly identified role for all those assessing and supporting post-registration students. Thus any support offered to students is over and above the full-time responsibilities of the community learning disability nurse, as it is for most mentors supporting community specialist practitioner students.

Community learning disability nurse (CLDN) students are taught with students from other disciplines and the standards of assessment of practice are the same for all. It follows that mentors must have the same opportunities for role preparation as other groups in order to ensure that the facilitation of learning, teaching and assessing is both equitable and comparable.

The issues of significance for CLDNs include mentors' educational needs, the viability of programmes for students and continuity of the mentor role. In addition the issues of placements and assessment of the student both need consideration.

Viability of programmes

The ENB (1998) highlight that with regards to the specialist practitioner award CLDN, 'it is perceived by some that the numbers may be too small to be viable'. Certainly I could reinforce that programme viability is a problem, as over the last three years each cohort at the Manchester Metropolitan University has attracted fewer than ten, including students undertaking the course on a full and part-time basis. Viability of the CLDN programme is not just one of applicants with the appropriate qualifications, it is also an issue of appropriately qualified mentors able to support students in practice. The problem for the mentor is one of continuity of experience. If students from one team undertake the CLDN award on an annual basis, then a bank of appropriately qualified mentors can be developed and maintained. However, many CLDN teams send a student in one year but not in subsequent years, so there is no 'pool' of qualified practitioners and little opportunity to develop the mentor profile within a team.

The preparation of the mentor

In the past some CLDN teams have supported the academic development of their staff whilst others have focused on service-led professional development. Thus currently some teams have a full complement of CLDNs whilst other teams have no staff with that qualification. CLDN is one area where nurses can be working in the specialism, and indeed take up senior positions, without necessarily holding a specialist community qualification. Thus as Jukes (1994a) highlights, this 'affords managers of services ... the soft option of employing RNMHs without a specialist community nursing qualification'.

Many of those nurses who hold the CLDN qualification studied when the award was at certificate or diploma level. It is unclear how many of these nurses have undertaken further study to gain a diploma or degree. Culley and Genders (1999), in a study of the role of community learning disability nurses in supporting parents who have a learning disability, highlighted that of their study of 266 nurses just over a third held the CLDN qualification and only 16% held a diploma. There is no indication that any of these 266 CLDNs held degree level qualifications or post-graduate awards. This suggests that CLDNs have some way to go to achieve sufficient mentors at degree level and above to support students undertaking the specialist practitioner award.

With small teams of few nurses the only way to provide effective support and assessment for CLDN specialist practitioner students is to plan ahead. It is important to prepare mentors this year to support the student of next year.

A community team is planning to send one of their members of staff onto the specialist practitioner award in CLD nursing. However, there are no qualified mentors in the team and whilst team members have appropriate academic qualifications, e.g. degree level or masters level study, none of the team members hold a community nursing qualification.

In other local teams there are nurses with appropriate professional quali-fications, i.e. the ENB 805/806/807 CLDN qualifications, but who lack degree and in some cases diploma level qualifications.

Case study 12.1 Mentorship requirements: who and where?

In this situation flexible means of supporting the student must be found and the specialist award leader from the HEI will need to ensure close contact with the mentor and student to provide the necessary support. I would suggest there are a number of strategies that could be adopted:

(1) A nurse within the team who does not hold the usual qualifications *exceptionally* takes on the role of mentor
(2) An 'out of area' placement is found for the student
(3) An 'out of area' mentor is found to support the student in the student's 'home' team.

In option (1) it may be possible to assess the suitability of a named nurse within the team who can undertake the role. Criteria for approving such a person must be in place, for example time in post, professional role and responsibilities, professional skills and attributes and other expertise in edu-cating students such as pre-registration, social work or other student groups. It must be made explicit that this is a one-off situation and that members of staff must gain the necessary skills (academic and/or professional) to undertake the role of mentor in the future. The ENB (1998) report on learning disability practice placements highlights very clearly that it is the responsibility of the education provider (the HEI) to 'ensure that practice placements meet the Board's standards' and a part of the audit of placements will be an audit of mentor qualifications. The ENB officer undertaking annual monitoring review ensures that these standards are met. Thus the exceptional nature of this mentor role must be acknowledged and education issues addressed by the community team.

If option (2) in the above list is chosen it must be clear from the start who will pay for this 'out of area' supported placement and the expertise of the mentor. Locally the workforce development Confederation pay replacement costs and thus if the team can make a short-term appointment then the service will not be adversely affected by an out of area placement. A contract must also be set up to ensure the student has access to an appropriate client case-load. This is a similar situation to that experienced by local students under-taking the health visiting award, i.e. the student has a contract with the out of area team for the duration of the course.

The final option (3) of 'buying in' the services of an appropriately qualified mentor may be an easier option than an out of area placement. Here the student will already hold a contract with their seconding team. However, buying in an expert results in support from a distance rather than the support that many students receive 'over the desk'. An agreed timetable between the mentor and the student is needed to ensure that the necessary support is available. Regular meetings to discuss progress and address issues are needed. The opportunity for the mentor to observe the student undertaking a range of activities is also vital to ensuring the student's competence in assessed areas. A problem with an arrangement of this nature is that the mentor may not know the resources available in the student's local area and thus the additional support of a local nurse mentor knowledgeable about the local resources may also be necessary.

Support for the mentor

The models of student support for exceptional situations raise issues of support for the mentor. One may suggest that the support needs of a new mentor in CLDN are similar to other new mentors. They need a colleague they can shadow or a peer for support. However, many CLDN work within small teams with few appropriately qualified nurses, so the problem may be a lack of professional peer support resulting in professional isolation for the mentor. The ENB (2000, p.5) point out that 'the formal structures . . . that support peer interaction no longer exist' for learning disability nurses and thus they advocate networking.

If few opportunities for mentor support exist in a team then mentors must use the support offered by the HEI. Regular meetings are essential to highlight the issues and look at mechanisms for addressing them. The opportunity to share knowledge and expertise is vital. Whilst it is valuable for CLDN mentors to meet as a group they can also learn from and gain support from mentors from other disciplines. In addition to those meetings, visits to placements by the specialist award leader allow the essential one-to-one support. In some situations these meetings and visits may be more frequent than is usual, to support the mentor rather than to address student issues. Alternative mechanisms of support in the form of a CLD forum do exist and mentors are advised to access those in their locality.

In addition to the formal and informal support discussed above, mentors are also recommended to access the mentor preparation that is available in the HEI.

The student as learner

The variety of learning disability nursing students entering a specialist practitioner award course is vast. The student may already be a community nurse but equally may come from the residential sector. The student may be newly qualified or have many years of experience. The student may be senior to their mentor in terms of grade.

The manager of a learning disability nursing team applies to undertake the CLDN course but only nurses whom s/he manages are appropriately qualified to undertake the role of mentor. The question here is who should take on the role of mentor and what support will that mentor require?

Assuming that the mentor will be an appropriately qualified member of the team, an important starting point for the mentor is to acknowledge that the manager of the service is taking on a new role, that of CLDN student, and is gaining total or partial release from the role of manager. Both specialist student (manager) and mentor (team member) must acknowledge the different role. Facilitation of learning and assessment requires an honest and critical evaluation of an individual. If the mentor feels that this is impossible because of the previous relationship then s/he should not mentor the student. The specialist award leader should liaise with the service manager to identify someone else to undertake that role.

Case study 12.2 Managing potential role and relationship conflict

Many learning disability nurses enter specialist practitioner award programmes from the team that they return to as students. It is possible that the mentor and student may have worked collaboratively in the past or have provided one another with supervision. There is the potential for a previous close working relationship between two peers getting in the way of the current role of mentor and student.

The variety of students in CLDN provides the mentor with a challenge. The practice experience must be appropriate for the student to ensure they benefit from the course regardless of their starting point. Given the variety of CLDN students, each student will experience a different journey through the course as his or her previous skills and knowledge will influence that journey. However, the outcome must be the same for all students – a specialist practitioner in community learning disability nursing. Therefore each student must have specific learning objectives that allow their individual development of skills and knowledge. It is important that the mentor acknowledges the uniqueness of each student and helps the student to set pertinent objectives taking into consideration the student's past experience and knowledge.

Harding and Greig (1994) highlight the importance of selection and preparation of the mentor. However, the continuing support of the mentor by both the service and the HEI is vital to assure that *effective* facilitation of teaching, learning and assessment will occur and that the mentor can carry out all elements of their role simultaneously.

The key to facilitation of appropriate learning experiences in all situations is the professionalism of the mentor and the student. It is important that the mentor sets the boundaries, arranges to meet regularly and is honest and clear in their feedback (see Chapter 8). Where there is a change of role, the mentor needs to discuss this at the first student-teacher meeting to set boundaries (see Chapter 6). It may also be valuable to put in place other strategies that help to put a line under the previous relationship. For example, it may be possible or essential for the student to move to a different team or base.

Clearly a learning contract will help to form the relationship of mentor and student. An early meeting with student, mentor and university teacher to set up an agreed contract will allow all parties to focus on the issues that are important to the CLDN student's development and allow assessment of those areas in practice.

Student learning – environment, experience and assessment

If one is to provide a quality learning environment there are a number of factors that need consideration. The issue of competition of placements is as great in CLDN as in other areas. The ENB (1998) point out that the unusual feature of CLDN is that at both pre- and post-registration most educational opportunities are offered in the community. Thus the demand for community-based support by a mentor is great. However, added to this pressure on mentors is the fact that many of the learning disability placement opportunities are in non-health provision. Work in the social services sector, private sector, education sector and the 'not-for-profit' organisations makes up a large percentage of the case load (ENB 1998) and thus when this practice is provided elsewhere the challenge for mentors is teaching, learning and assessment in a range of settings.

Jukes (1994b, p.851), in a review of supervisory systems for CLDN, highlights that there is 'a lack of commitment ... in relation to supervision of practice'. Given the variety of settings in which the student may practise, the mentor will experience difficulty in supervising all aspects of practice but must provide the commitment to supervise that practice. The key issue must be to gain a fair assessment of the student who is working in this wide range of settings. Critical discourse (Chapter 8), clinical supervision (Chapter 6) and a reflective diary may provide valuable evidence on which to base an assessment. Equally the views of others are important but the mentor must exercise critical evaluation of others' assessments of the student. The non-NHS sector employs few nurses (ENB 1998) and other professional groups may have differing expectations of CLDN students.

The multi-disciplinary nature of the learning environment may have problems for the mentor but it does have strengths for the CLDN student. It provides the breadth of experience that a specialist practitioner student needs to ensure effective liaison and work with other professionals; if used well it provides a wide learning experience for the student.

Student assessment

The issue of passing or failing a student is always difficult but when the person you are assessing is a colleague or indeed a manager the task becomes more difficult. Most CLDN students, whether they pass or fail, will be returning to the team where they experience their practice. It is therefore essential that the mentor gains the necessary education and support to make even the most difficult decisions about a student.

Effective student assessment relies on the mentor being academically able to assess students in practice. The work of Culley and Genders (1999) suggests that few CLDNs have the necessary academic qualifications to effectively assess students at degree level. Given that 'the assessment of community nursing practice is dependent on the expertise of the community practice teachers [mentors] who are gatekeepers to the profession' (Goding 1997a p. 161), it is imperative that managers ensure that mentors are supported to undertake preparation and continuing study to support their role.

Harding and Greig (1994) discuss the role of the practice assessor of pre-registration students and emphasise tripartite accountability. They consider that the practice assessor (mentor) must be accountable to the learner, to him or herself and to the HEI who in essence contract the mentor to undertake that role. This tripartite arrangement should be exploited by the CLDN mentor to ensure all are involved in the process and also to ensure that all gain the support from the other parties involved.

Conclusion

If CLDNs are to achieve the same status as other community practitioner groups then their managers must ensure the education of their workforce. As Clifton *et al.* (1993, p.17) quite rightly said 'clients and their carers have the right to expect appropriately qualified professionals to realise their total needs'. Jukes (1994b) points out 'training should be supported and acknowledged by the government, the UKCC and the National Boards as an essential requirement for practice'. Jukes is referring to CLDN courses but one could argue the same for all mentors.

The challenge is to ensure that mentors in the field of CLDN have the same educational standards as those in other areas of nursing. They need to take up the opportunities of further education for themselves and to ensure that the students they support and assess gain the best possible experience. A further key challenge for the mentor is to ensure that they gain quality support whilst undertaking their role.

Chapter 13
Community Children's Nursing

Carole Proud

As Carole Proud points out, community children's nursing is developing rapidly, with the majority of mentors being new to the role. Carole's study of mentors has enabled her to provide a chapter that illuminates how appropriate mentoring can be organised for students from a wide variety of backgrounds and with different prior experiences.

Introduction

Children have always been cared for at home; parents have attempted, and always will, to meet the needs of their sick or disabled child. In the past professional nursing input was rarely required. For, as Bishop (2000, p.164) noted:

> 'Caring is not the prerogative of nurses – many people can care and be the advocate. It is the provision of professional and knowledgeable care that differentiates nurses.'

The knowledge required to care for the sick child is changing. The pattern of childhood illness has altered, childhood mortality rates are falling and more children are surviving into adulthood with the burden of chronic illness, 'technically dependent' or with a life limiting disorder (Botting 1995). Furthermore, there is now an acceptance of the value of home care and an acknowledgement of the rights of the child (Franklin 1995) to expert support. These factors have led to a rapid rise in the number of community children's nursing (CCN) teams within the UK (Muir & Sidey 2000). The teams are welcomed by the children, parents and professionals but for the children's nurses working within them there has been a tremendous struggle to develop a philosophy of care, a knowledge base for practice and clinical protocols. For example, Kirk and Glendinning (1998) explored the tensions in the relationship between community nurses and carers, and the particular issue of 'parent as carer'. They suggested that these concerns need to be addressed if appropriate help and support is to be offered to families.

As the newly formed CCN teams work to establish their role, the UKCC (1994, 1998) called for the establishment of discrete specialist routes into children's community nursing. The CCN practitioners were asked to extend their skills further and take on a new role, that of a mentor. Five years later, a group of CCN mentors reflected on their thoughts and experiences of 'taking students'.

The intention of this chapter is to explore the specific challenges of being a mentor in community children's nursing. The themes are derived from a focus group session with six community children's nursing (CCN) mentors who have worked to establish the CCN course at the University of Northumbria at Newcastle.

Focus group

Krueger (1994) examined the value of focus groups in profit-making orga- nisations and the public sector. He felt that the strength of the focus group was in the debate and discussion engendered by the facilitators' questions. In this group the CCNs knew each other, were passionate about the value of home care for children and talked freely about their experiences of mentoring from the initial request to perform the role to the final assessment of the student. In analysing the data four distinct themes arose:

- Uncertainty as a practice teacher – have I the skills?
- Different students – different experiences
- Helping students cope with uncertainty
- Making judgements – the assessment process.

Uncertainties as a mentor – have I the skills?

This was seen in the comment:

> 'I knew I had to offer that first placement to T, there was no one else and we need CCNs with the specialist practitioner qualification. But I was scared. I don't have a degree and, at that time, I hadn't a mentoring qualification.'
> (CCN 1)

When the first cohort of students commenced their course, the university had a very small group of practitioners to call upon for support. Indeed, this was not unique to the University of Northumbria, Neill and Muir acknowledging the national concerns in accessing placements in 1997. However, we did have an extremely motivated group of practitioners. It was Proctor *et al.* (1999) who wrote of the 'pioneering spirits' amongst the CCNs who were acting flexibly and creatively to meet the challenges of their new role. In examining the 'individualised careers' of CCNs, Proctor referred to studies of the careers of teachers where early concerns are for survival and identification, running into competence concerns as 'the job starts to fit', and ultimately into concern for personal extension, influence on organisations and impact on clients. The first CCN mentors at UNN showed both the 'pioneering spirit' and the wish to extend their practice further. To facilitate the practitioners in their work with students a support package was developed, which included:

- Encouragement and priority in attending a formal mentor's programme of study
- Individual and group support to understand curriculum and assessment
- Tripartite approach, whereby the university teacher, mentor and student met together to examine issues from practice.

One of the main themes of this 'support package' was to highlight the value given to 'practice-based' knowledge by the course team, the need to facilitate practice-based experiences for the student and to work with the student to uncover the theory which underpins it. Nyiri examined this concept of practical knowledge and expertise stating (1988, pp. 20–21):

'One becomes an expert not simply by absorbing explicit knowledge of the type found in textbooks, but through experience, that is, through repeated trials, "failing, succeeding, wasting time and effort-getting to feel the problem, learning to go by the book and when to break the rules". Human experts gradually absorb a "repertory of working rules of thumb", or "heuristics", that, combined with book knowledge, make them "expert practitioners". This practical, heuristic knowledge, as attempts to simulate it on the machine have shown, is "hardest to get at because experts – or anyone else – rarely have the self-awareness to recognise what it is. So it must be mined out of their heads painstakingly, one jewel at a time".'
(Quotes in this extract from Feigenbaum & McCorduck, 1984)

More recently CCN mentors have been encouraged to extend their practice and reflect further, by either entering masters programmes or considering gaining 'academic points' through practice development, i.e. accreditation of work based learning (AWBL).

From her initial position of concern, CCN 1 noted:

'I really enjoyed having T as a student – she made me think about practice and I discovered the value of reflection – I learnt a lot.'

Different students – different experiences

The CCN mentors recognised and commented on the tremendous number of variables in fitting a student to a practice placement. The students were all registered children's nurses but their experience was vast: some had community experience and had worked as district nurses or health visitors, others had a very specialist background in oncology or cystic fibrosis care, whilst other students joined the course with ward management experience in general paediatrics. At the same time, the models of CCN practice were diverse. Winter and Teare (1997) classified CCN services into four models, distinguishing between generalist and specialist services and whether they were based in acute or community NHS Trusts.

In linking students to placement areas, a personal profile of the student was established, then a dialogue occurred between student, manager, mentor and lecturer to determine the 'best fit' placement. Placements varied tremendously.

Jenny was employed in a general paediatric ward as a G grade sister. She had diverse and up-to-date skills in acute paediatric care – her long-term aim was to develop a children's nursing outreach service from the ward on which she worked. The challenge was to support her in developing her understanding and philosophy of community care and primary care teams. In the first semester it was decided that Jenny would work with an experienced health visitor who was also a mentor. The health visitor worked within an integrated nursing team, and the primary care team had a strong commitment to child health. For the rest of the course, Jenny worked with the CCN team, which supported children and families with special needs across the city; many of these children were already well known to Jenny from work.

Case study 13.1 Specific placements to meet learning needs: example 1

Tim had gained his RN/DipHE (child) qualification ten years earlier. Since qualifying he had worked as a children's nurse in Saudi Arabia for five years. On returning to the UK he started work as a school nurse within the local community trust. In the evening he studied for a law degree. Tim identified the need for a CCN service to support children with life limiting disorders in the community and was appointed to lead the service. It was decided that Tim needed to refocus on paediatric systems and procedures in the area. One of the cystic fibrosis specialist nurses was also a qualified district nurse; she took on the role of mentor and facilitated a range of experiences for Tim within her specialist team and with the diabetic and oncology teams. To supplement this experience Tim spent a fortnight with a well-established CCN team in another part of the country.

Case study 13.2 Specific placements to meet learning needs: example 2

These diverse experiences and diverse opportunities led to diverse placements. As one CCN mentor commented:

> 'To prepare me for the CCN role I had qualified as an adult district nurse; I spent the year totally frustrated that I rarely saw a child. "Knitting" placements so that they meet the needs of the student just makes sense.'
>
> (CCN 2)

Fundamental to this approach is the establishment of a learning contract between the student and the mentor, generally with input from the university teacher. Many writers have explored the value of contracts in promoting individual centred learning (Reed & Proctor 1993; Lowry 1997), although it was Schön (1987, p.167) who classically established the argument that:

'Building a relationship conducive to learning begins with the explicit or implicit establishment of a contract that sets expectations for a dialogue: what will coach and student give to and get from each other? Further, how will they be accountable to each other.'

One CCN mentor noted:

'Learning contracts were essential ... we all know each other in children's nursing, R already worked in our team – we were friends. It helped to re-establish our roles as mentor and student'.

(CCN 3)

Helping students cope with uncertainty

The CCN mentors understood the complexity of their role. To the question 'What do CCN students need to know for practice?', CCN 3 responded:

'If it was just technical procedures like gastrostomy feeds or giving IV antibiotics it would be easy but it's the other things – you get to know families, you know when they're worn out and can't get respite care. Last week, one mum had just heard her 'well' son had been found with drugs at school – she blamed herself because she's always busy with T. How do you help students understand that side of the work?'

CCN 4:

'For some families it's OK giving IVs or changing tubes, but not for others. How do you help students work out what is really happening in families?'

These very positive examples clearly demonstrate the mentors' understanding of the complexities of care management. Care management is based on the therapeutic relationship between family and nurse, resource issues, the 'power' struggles within the 'multi-disciplinary team', local and national politics as well as the evidence base which underlies the task to be performed. For the mentor to address the issues of uncertainty and complexity with her student it is valuable to draw upon different social theories (Fox 1999). Ghaye *et al.* (2000) would argue that nurses need to consider, if not embrace, the postmodern theories of Foucault, Lyotard and Guattari to enable them to understand the everyday ethical dilemmas within practice.

Very simply, postmodern theorists question our reliance on scientific knowledge and rationality, which emerged with the 'enlightenment'. They acknowledge the uncertainty and contradiction in an unpredictable world and suggest that the main basis for the legitimisation of knowledge is its relevance and usefulness to practice. The art of community children's nursing, the flexibility and creativity emerge from the freedom to explore and analyse practice. The mentor is in a key position to facilitate this analysis.

The everyday strategies to explore practice include:

- Use of reflective frameworks
- Critical incident technique
- Analysis of discourse/narratives from practice
- Promoting a multi-disciplinary approach to problem solving
- Learning culture.

Some of these techniques are examined in more detail in Chapters 5 and 7 of the text.

On a less theoretical and more practical base, Proctor *et al.* (1999) discussed the key skills required by CCNs. Their account is based on research with families and practitioners and acknowledges the problems of defining a role 'which is currently characterised by variation and contrast' (p.98). Six key skills are discussed:

- Formal knowledge/technical skills
- Skills for managing their own work
- Relational, interpersonal and support skills
- Co-ordinating knowledge and skills
- Teaching skills
- Thinking skills.

These skills are used to suggest a process model of the curriculum where consensus knowledge (knowledge which is technical and 'currently' indisputable) and indeterminate knowledge (knowledge derived from areas of philosophy) coexist to equip the practitioner to cope with the challenges and uncertainty of practice. In this way the mentor is able to help the student develop the skills and creativity required for practice, practice which changes and develops with time and context.

Making judgements – assessing students

The issues around assessment are considered in Chapter 8. However, for CCN mentors the assessment process caused significant anxiety: 'My greatest concern was the assessment form' (CCN 4).

This concern appeared to be heightened by issues specific to CCN practice:

- Relationship between the student and mentor. Children's nursing is a small area of practice and the mentor frequently knew the student as a colleague/friend.
- 'Newness' of the area of practice – the mentors were new to their role and

were still developing their own ideologies of practice. Would they be able to recognise safe and ultimately 'specialist' practice?

Accepting these difficulties, we looked at how we could support mentors by developing networks and examining strategies to facilitate the assessment process. The networks aimed to promote 'learning conversations' between mentors so that together they learned and explored the expectations of the course and the specific challenges of the assessment process. In practice, they met together at monthly 'regional CCN forum' meetings and at regular meetings arranged at the university. Individual support by university teachers was also available for mentors in the practice setting. The opportunity to share experiences proved valuable for mentors and university teachers.

Reed and Proctor (1993, p.179) state that:

'Assessment is primarily a judgemental exercise, in which the assessor must judge whether the assessee has passed or failed according to pre-determined criteria.'

The CCN mentors highlighted the strategies which they found useful in assisting them to make judgements about students:

- Use of learning contracts (Lowry 1997) – as well as setting content they also allowed the mentor to clarify role expectation with the student. The concept of a professional, supportive relationship can be established and the methods and timing of assessment negotiated.
- Formative assessment (Jarvis & Gibson 1997) – an early, diagnostic assessment that is shared with the student. It was found useful in enabling the mentor to change/amend the learning contract to meet the student's needs and, if necessary, to seek support at an early stage in the placement.
- Self-assessment (Jarvis & Gibson 1997) – seen as a particularly valuable method of assessment because of the close relationship between the mentor and student and the wish to encourage self-reflection in the student. As one mentor commented:

'It was useful because it really made me stop and listen to how the student saw her progress and the value of the experiences she had undertaken . . . It let us focus on how we would alter things for the next semester.

(CCN 2)

- Partnership between university teachers and mentors – in determining the assessment criteria for practice the CCN mentors are fully involved so that the assessment reflects the reality of practice.

As mentors gain experience in working with and assessing students they are able to support practitioners taking on the role for the first time, in many ways acting as a 'critical friend'.

Conclusion

Fundamental to this chapter is the fact that community children's nursing is a relatively new area of nursing practice. Working with the CCNs and listening to their narratives has helped to highlight their specific philosophies of care and their unique way of working to support families with a sick or disabled child in the community. When the CCNs were asked to support students who wished to undertake the specialist practitioner award, they were faced with a further series of challenges. The challenges centred around insecurities about their own emerging practice, their skills as a mentor, understanding 'specialist practice' and the logistics of how to make space for more activities and roles. However, as student and mentor have worked together, exploring issues from practice and developing practice-based initiatives for the ENB Higher Award, the community children's nurses have begun to talk about the maturing of their practice and the reflective strategies which have promoted learning – for the student and themselves. The next five years for CCN mentors will, hopefully, be a time of consolidation and reappraisal. However, further challenges exist in the form of nurse prescribing, *Making a Difference* (DoH 1999a), the impact of the The Human Rights Act 1998 and perhaps more, which all need to be assimilated into practice.

Chapter 14

Health Visiting

Joanna Bateman

In health visiting there are many areas of responsibility where specialist practitioner students require the facilitation of learning courtesy of an expert practitioner. Invariably the majority of health visiting students are 'new' and yet (normally) must reach fruition at the same time as all students undertaking the same course of education. Joanna Bateman provides the mentor with strategies for enabling constant student development so that students can move from novice to specialist practitioner with plenty of challenges but minimal headache.

Introduction

This chapter provides an overview of some of the issues which mentors who facilitate health visiting students are likely to encounter. The challenge for mentors is to facilitate students' progress from 'novice', with most students having had little experience of health visiting prior to the course, to specialist practitioner in a course that could be as short as 32 weeks. This chapter will focus on the journey students take, in learning a new role and for many adopting a new philosophy.

The last few years have seen changes to the educational preparation of students on the health visiting programme, as well as exciting opportunities for the profession to become involved in public health work and work collaboratively to address health inequalities. Government documents are naming health visitors as the profession central to many initiatives (Home Office 1998; DoH 1999ab), and students in the early 2000s have the opportunity of an exciting career ahead of them. The challenge for the mentor is to prepare them for this new and diverse role.

This chapter will discuss some current issues in health visiting practice, and then consider aspects related to teaching, learning and assessing in health visiting. It is recognised that health visiting practice and health visitor-client interactions are complex, and this can pose difficulties for both the teaching and assessing of practice. It is not the purpose of this chapter to provide a blueprint for the teaching and assessing of health visiting students, but rather to raise some of these issues and encourage the reader to consider the relevance of these to their practice setting.

Health visiting: some current issues and dilemmas for mentors

Recent government policy documents have outlined plans for health visiting which would enable the profession to move forward into a wider public health role, and health visiting has been described as being 'at the crossroads' (McMahon 2000) with many exciting opportunities open to it. Health visitors are being encouraged to adopt a 'family-centred public health role' by recommendations in *Making A Difference* (DoH 1999a, p.61) and *Our Healthier Nation* (DoH 1999b), and details of this are given in Fig. 14.1. However, there remains a 'policy-practice gap', with GP attachment, the current focus on primary care and in some areas the legacy of GP fund holding, meaning that much practice is still individually focused on general practitioner clients. There is now a need for health visitors to embrace the concepts of public health and shift from the current emphasis on individuals and families to populations and communities (McMahon 2000), although it is recognised that the current system of GP attachment may hamper this approach. Many practitioners find it difficult to define public health, and research has suggested that public health work still takes second place to the 'bread and butter' of health visiting practice (Pearson *et al.* 2000). However, the role of nurses and health visitors in public health is an area of considerable interest: the Health Development Agency is currently auditing skills required for public health, and the Department of Health were due to distribute a public health tool kit for health visitors in early 2001.

Mentors have a difficult role here in that they need to ensure that students not only gain the skills required to fulfil the health visitor's role of today but also have the skills required to take practice forward. This is not helped by the lack of a clear model of effective health visiting or vision of health visiting in the future (McMahon 2000). It may be useful for mentors to refer to the model

---

- 'Deliver child health programmes and work in partnership with families to develop and agree tailored health plans to address their parenting and health needs;
- Run parenting groups and provide home visits to help improve support, advice and information to parents – and especially to vulnerable children and their families – supporting initiatives such as Sure Start;
- Work through Primary Care Groups to identify the health needs of neighbourhoods and special groups such as the homeless, and agree local health plans;
- Work with local communities to help them identify and tackle their own health needs, such as measures to combat the social isolation of elderly people or the development of local accident prevention schemes;
- Provide health promotion programmes to target accidents, cancer, mental health, coronary heart disease and stroke.'

Fig. 14.1 Family-centred public health role for health visitors (Department of Health (1999a, pp.61–2)).

for health visiting described by McMahon (2000), or the 'universal health visiting service' outlined by Robotham (2000), and use these as a guide to ensure that students gain a broad perspective of health visiting during the course. Diverse skills are required to meet the health needs of individuals, families and communities, and skills in health needs analysis, empowerment, advocacy, collaboration and multi-agency working are essential if health visiting is truly to adopt the public health agenda.

A likely shortfall of health visitors in around 2005–2010 (McMahon 2000) requires health visitors to re-examine the nature of their practice and explore new ways of working. This shortfall is caused by the current age profile of the health visiting profession, with a high proportion due to retire shortly, and the reduction in the numbers of students entering training in the 1990s. Health visiting practice will have to change, and it is anticipated that in the future health visitors will take a more active role in leading skill mix teams (DoH 1999b). Adopting a skill mix approach would enable health visitors to delegate some 'routine' work and adopt a wider public health approach. It is important that the mentor considers the implications of this for students, who have to develop the skills required to lead a health visiting team in a much-shortened course.

Recent changes in specialist practitioner education present additional demands on the mentor. Until the new nursing, midwifery and health visitor training rules (Statutory Instrument 2000 no. 2554) were passed in the summer of 2000, the new shortened courses were at odds with the statutory instrument in terms of entry requirement, length of course and underlying philosophy (Cowley *et al.* 2000). The new statutory instrument (UKCC 2000b) will enable students to enter the specialist practitioner award of health visiting from many different backgrounds (Parts 1, 3, 5, 8, 10, 12, 13, 14 or 15 of the register), and direct entry midwives are now able to train as health visitors. This widening of the entry gates to health visiting will affect the role of the mentor, as students will enter the programme with wide variations in their skills, knowledge and experience, and a flexible and adaptable approach to their education is essential. With the increasing use of staff nurses in skill mix teams, there may also be more experienced practitioners entering the course in the future.

Many students, especially those who have come from working within a particularly medical model, find that they have to 'un-learn' part of their previous role. This can be a particular challenge for mentors, who must ensure that the student understands the role and principles underpinning health visiting (Twinn & Cowley 1992), and the difference between health visiting and their previous role. At the time of writing there is debate about whether only a nursing background can provide the skills and attributes required for health visiting, or indeed whether a nursing background does provide these skills and attributes. A report has suggested a pilot project to assess the feasibility of a multi-professional group of students at post-graduate level, and also a direct entry degree programme (Cowley *et al.* 2000).

It is not possible to discuss here the many other factors that affect the role of health visitors, although it is acknowledged that widening inequalities in health, expansion of Sure Start programmes, the increasing proportion of elderly people, the expansion of nurse prescribing, and Government policy such as National Service Frameworks and *The NHS Plan* (DoH 2000a) will influence the future role and direction that health visiting takes. However, the real future and direction of the health visiting profession lies with health visitors themselves: there is a need to define an effective model of health visiting practice, and strong leadership is required by professional bodies and key players (including mentors) to take this model forward.

Managing the learning experience

The learning environment

Although the skills and attributes of the mentor are fundamental to facilitating effective learning, it is also important that both the health visiting and primary health care team are committed to providing a suitable learning environment and have some awareness of the course and learning needs of the health visitor student. Recent years have seen many changes to the way health visitor case-loads have been organised (including geographical allocation, GP attachment, and corporate case-loads), and with the current focus on public health it is possible that practitioners will identify more closely with a specific community in the future. It is important that the mentor analyses the strengths and weaknesses of the practice placement, in terms of preparing a student for practice anywhere in the country and not just the local area. An 'ideal' placement area would provide a mix of client groups, but inequalities that exist across the country mean that some students will be placed in areas of extreme poverty, and others in areas of affluence. Here in the north-west region, with the highest illness and mortality rates in England (Flynn & Knight 1998), many students report being distressed at seeing the poverty and deprivation that exist and mentors should try and prepare them for this. As case study 14.1 demonstrates, different areas provide students with diverse learning experiences.

Catherine – placement area is predominately middle class, good attendance rates for clinics and few no-access visits. She feels challenged by clients – needs to have read the paper daily, watched *Newsnight* on television, accessed the web etc. Learns good 'basic' health visiting skills. Feels apprehensive about dealing with child protection and has had no experience of this on placement, but has attended training and discussed this with her mentor at length.

Fiona – placement is an inner city area and the case-load contains a large percentage of vulnerable families. Two child protection issues arose in the first few weeks of placement, and she has observed case-conferences and core-group meetings. Has experience of Sure Start and community development initiatives, and good awareness of the health needs of ethnic minority clients. Feels apprehensive about dealing with challenges posed by clients in a more affluent area.

Case study 14.1 Students' experience of very different placements

Diversity of practice is important, and large teams of health visitors, shared offices and integrated nursing teams all have their advantages in terms of the experience offered to a student. Whilst students value the intense input from their mentor, they also require different perspectives on health visiting practice so they can model their own practice from a range of practitioners/styles. Mentors have a role to ensure that the placement experience offered provides a broad grounding in health visiting practice and enables students to meet the learning outcomes outlined by the ENB (1995) and the university. Whilst a formal period of alternative practice is no longer a requirement, it may be useful for students to spend time in other areas and this should be negotiated with the student. This is of course only proposed if the placement would enable the student to meet specific learning objectives that would not be met in the main placement area.

Teaching and learning in health visiting practice

The diversity of students' backgrounds certainly makes for interesting university discussions, and requires mentors to undertake a thorough assessment of the prior experience and needs of the student at the start of the course. It is important to acknowledge the students' past experience and build on their skills, whilst introducing the practice and philosophy of health visiting. The student has an important role in taking responsibility for their learning; however, it is difficult for those new to a professional role to state what they need to learn at the start of the course and some direction from the mentor is required. The programme must therefore be flexible and provide a range of experiences to meet the individual student's learning needs. A useful text for students in terms of practical advice relating to children and families is Booth and Luker (1999), and familiarity with this material should help their confidence early in the course. Students will probably find the texts by Appleton and Cowley (2000) and Robotham and Sheldrake (2000) more useful for the theoretical aspects of the course, with Craig and Lindsay's (2000) text providing a useful insight into nursing and public health.

Building a good relationship and preparing the student for feelings of de-skilling that frequently occur in the first few months of the course is crucial, and students require a considerable amount of support when making the transition to health visiting from their previous role (see case study 14.2). It is useful to discuss the change in philosophy and conceptual approach that health visiting requires, and Robotham and Sheldrake (2000) argue that rather than being de-skilled, the students are shifting from reductionism to holism in their role transition.

'The first few months of the course were awful and I wanted desperately to go back to my old job where I felt secure, knowledgeable and was competently in charge of a ward. How things have changed ... I feel unable to deal with the many questions we get asked on visits. My mentor is really understanding and says this is normal, but right now I feel really de-skilled and that I cannot contribute anything to clients I meet.'

Case study 14.2 The first few months of the placement

The one-to-one student-mentor relationship can be intense and stressful for both parties (Jardine & Asherton 1992), and in health visiting this is particularly likely to be an issue due to the new role the student has to learn and the complex and sensitive nature of much of the work. Many mentors organise peer support groups or hold regular meetings to discuss educational issues, and support for students in the form of clinical supervision can be helpful.

Students on the health visiting programme will be expected to critically evaluate practice, consider the potential effectiveness of the role of the health visitor and ensure that their practice is evidence-based. It is therefore likely that they will challenge existing practice, and the health visiting team should welcome the opportunity for this debate. Initially, many students can appear to be overly critical about practice not being 'research-based' and perhaps not appreciate the importance of practice-based evidence. This can be due to their lack of practice-based knowledge and experience, and their reliance on knowledge from research papers and theoretical sources (such as the recent systematic review into the effectiveness of domiciliary health visiting (Elkan *et al.* 2000)). The mentor has a fundamental role in enabling the student to integrate theory into practice and, drawing on practical experience, to put theory into perspective. Intuitive knowledge is also important in health visiting practice (Goding & Cain 1999; Ling & Luker 2000), and will be discussed later in relation to child protection issues.

An important element of the mentor's role is ensuring that the student not only learns the practical aspects required, but adopts an empowering approach and works in partnership with clients. Many students report feelings of frustration regarding their inability to 'solve' or 'help' with complex social problems, and anticipation of this by the mentor is useful, perhaps feeding into debate about empowerment and the principles underpinning health visiting practice (Twinn & Cowley 1992). It is not uncommon for students to feel disillusioned with society and the Government when working in very deprived areas, although since the recent formation of Health Action Zones and implementation of Sure Start programmes, student feedback is becoming more positive that something is starting to be done at a grass-roots level. Those fortunate enough to be placed in such areas should gain excellent experience of multi-agency working and collaboration.

In health visiting, the novice practitioner has to gain knowledge and skills in the 'basics' of health visiting, and then quickly move on to operate at the level described by Hudson and Forester (1995) which involves working independently supporting single clients, families and communities, in a complex interaction of social influences.

In view of the short length of the course, mentors have to expose students to complex situations early, in order for them to reach the learning outcomes for the programme. However, many of these skills will only be fully developed towards the end of the course or once qualified. Mentors should not expect students to be expert practitioners, but aim for a competent and safe practitioner (ENB 1995; UKCC 1998) who is able to fulfil the specialist practitioner role and is aware of their limitations.

It is important that the mentor emphasises the need to be flexible and client centred, as the unpredictability of health visiting can be difficult for students, especially where they specifically prepare for a visit only to find that the client's agenda is very different to theirs. Anecdotally many students report feelings of panic when, for the first time, a visit did not go according to their carefully rehearsed plan, and mentors should prepare students for this situation. Indeed, Cowley's research (1995) suggested that health visitors adopted:

> 'an approach to health promotion which requires a highly developed ability to cope in a safe and therapeutic way with shifting, uncertain and ill-defined health needs, and to recognise and respond to complex, potentially risk-filled situations.'

It is important that the demands placed on students entering this professional award and the complex skills required by health visitors are not underestimated.

Students will naturally compare their progress with each other, and whilst this can be useful when explored supportively, it can cause anxiety if they feel they are not progressing along with the group norm. Mentors often need to reassure students about variation in progress, and appreciate that no two students will progress from an observational role to supervised visits and then visiting unaccompanied at the same rate. It is vital that students have some control in their progression and feel confident to move on to the next stage, as student feedback frequently indicates that they visited too early by themselves and would have benefited from more supervised visits. Requirements in terms of 'case-load allocation' will vary across universities, but most courses now encourage students to take responsibility for families from early in the course and build both on numbers and complexity of cases as the course progresses. This mini caseload will be expanded gradually as the student develops, to a situation in 'consolidated practice' where they are expected to manage larger numbers of clients.

Child protection and domestic violence

Child protection and domestic violence are areas that many students are understandably anxious about, and previously it was recommended that students were not deliberately exposed to child protection issues or complex situations until later on in the course. However, with the reduction in both the length of the course and 'routine' visiting it is likely that exposure to vulnerable clients will come far earlier, as the focus of health visiting practice is on those in need. Training in child protection should take place prior to students undertaking any unaccompanied visits, so that at a minimum students are aware of the signs and symptoms of abuse and local child protection procedures. There have been many recent publications on domestic violence from both the Department of Health (2000d) and the Home Office (2000), and it is important that health visitors gain the skills and attributes necessary to work effectively with families affected by domestic violence. In view of the likely prevalence of domestic violence these skills are required for all practitioners, as there will be many clients suffering from domestic violence on every health visitor case-load in the country.

Using different sources of knowledge as a framework – authority, personal experience and intuition (Goding & Cain 1999) – some suggestions are made here as to how the mentor can facilitate learning about child protection and domestic violence, to complement the university input.

Authority

Students need to have a good awareness of research and reports on child protection and domestic violence, including risk factors, signs and symptoms, and Government policy or guidance. Publications such as the Health Visitors Association guide (HVA 1994), government documents (DoH/DfEE 1999; DoH 2000c; DoH 2000d), and local child protection policies are all fundamental to ensuring that students have a thorough knowledge base on the subject area. Assessing vulnerable families is an important element of the health visitor's role, and Appleton (1999) provides a useful overview of the subject area. The role of the mentor is to help integrate theory and practice, and encourage the integration of factual knowledge with other sources of knowledge, such as personal experience and intuition.

Personal experience

Students will be exposed to a wide variety of situations during the course, but may not necessarily be exposed to any known child abuse or domestic violence. Even if students do not gain any direct experience of working with vulnerable clients over the duration of the course, the mentor can prepare them for this role and ensure that they develop skills in observation, communication and critical reflection on practice. Students require the ability to learn from these personal experiences, and this should be facilitated by the mentor. The mentor also needs to explore the students' perceptions of what is acceptable in terms of treating children, women and other vulnerable groups such as the elderly. In view of the prevalence of child abuse and domestic violence, it is likely that some students entering health visiting will have been abused themselves, and it is important that these issues are explored sensitively and appropriate support given. Mentors need to ensure that students develop self-awareness and respond appropriately to any case of potential or actual abuse.

Intuition

An important element of health visiting knowledge is intuition or intuitive awareness (Goding & Cain 1999). Ling and Luker (2000) have recently researched intuition in the work of health visitors within child protection, and suggest that intuition is important for both the prevention and detection of abuse. Sensitivity and responsiveness are essential attributes, and Goding (1997b) believes these may be influenced by the practitioners' childhood experiences. As novice practitioners, students tend to doubt their intuition, especially where they may have different perspectives to their mentor. It is important that the role of intuition in health visiting practice is discussed with students and they are encouraged to verbalise and reflect on their feelings and develop their self-awareness.

Working with vulnerable families is a large element of many health visitors' roles, and mentors need to ensure that not only do students have the necessary knowledge and skills for this role, but that they consider their own safety as well as that of their clients. Some training should be provided on personal safety and risk assessment.

Assessment of practice

Whatever method the university uses, the assessment of practice in health visiting is complex and the role of the mentor in assessing students on this award should not be underestimated. Some of the learning outcomes for the specialist programme appear fairly straightforward to assess as they are based on the student being competent to undertake a practical task (e.g. undertaking health screening). However, for the majority of the learning outcomes the mentor is not just assessing the actual knowledge of the student or practical skills acquired, but their personal qualities and attitudes.

Indeed, Goding and Cain (1999) write about the nature of knowledge in health visiting practice and feel that:

> 'of equal (possibly greater) importance (than factual knowledge) is the individuality of the practitioner. If knowledge is to be effectively mediated to the client, she must be concerned, self-aware, possess specific capacities and qualities (for example, sensitivity and responsiveness), and have a disposition that is open and inquiring.'

Does this therefore mean that the mentor is required to assess the 'individuality' of the student? These characteristics are open to subjective interpretation, and in order to be fair to both the student and the profession they must be assessed as objectively as possible. Educational supervision for the mentor could be helpful with respect to any difficulties encountered in this area, and it is of course paramount that the mentor also possesses the attributes described above.

Students are also assessed on their ability to form and sustain relationships with clients. Whilst the mentor can observe and assess communication skills in terms of listening, non-verbal skills etc., the deeper issues in terms of what is happening within the relationship require more consideration. Practitioners who become over-involved with families (perhaps due to fear of rejection or a desire to 'help') can find it very difficult to be objective, and there are times when the practitioner's unmet needs are such that they become a 'helpaholic' (Dale *et al.* 1986). Not only does such an approach not fit with a model of empowerment, but more importantly in the context of child protection or domestic violence it could be the sign of a 'dangerous health visitor', who could engage in collusive relationships with clients (Dale *et al.* 1986). It is therefore important that the mentor encourages the student to be self-aware, explores the nature of relationships with clients and objectives for visits and interventions, and utilises all opportunities for critical reflection on practice. Mentors should be open and honest with students about the nature of their relationship with clients, and should spend time discussing such issues with students. There is no easy way of assessing such complex aspects of health visiting practice, and mentors require good observation and communication skills and the confidence to examine such issues in depth.

All aspects of assessment must be undertaken as objectively as possible, and any concerns articulated promptly and constructively to the student. One of the most difficult situations is where mentors state that they have a 'gut feeling' about a student, yet they may appear to be competent in terms of performing the visits according to Trust guidelines. These situations are far harder to deal with than when a student does not reach competencies in practical areas, yet with additional experience should do so. One example could be of a student who competently undertook visits, yet did not appear to be particularly interested in clients: a client's feedback stated that she appeared as if she was going through a process, rather than engaging with her. The mentor must clearly articulate to the student what the nature of the problem is, and what changes in attitude or performance are required. In all circumstances it is vital that concerns are voiced immediately, in order that appropriate support can be offered to the student, and the student is given the opportunity to develop. Clear communication and documentation is important and an action plan should be negotiated to address the issues. Mentors may require advice and support to deal with such difficult issues, and support from peers or managers can be useful. Involvement of the university teacher is essential in all situations where there is concern about the progress of a student.

Conclusion

Mentorship in health visiting is demanding, as students enter the award from a range of backgrounds with little experience in health visiting, and have to move from novice to specialist practitioner in one academic year. In view of the nature of much of health visiting, the assessment of practice can be difficult, as mentors will frequently be assessing personal attributes rather than practical skills. Objectivity is therefore fundamental and educational supervision for the mentor useful.

The health visiting profession is currently high on the Government agenda in relation to current policy documents (DoH 1999a,b), and there are opportunities to take health visiting forward to a new public health role. Mentors are at the forefront of practice, and have the challenge not only of ensuring that students are competent to undertake the current role but also of exposing them to the exciting practice of the future.

Chapter 15

Occupational Health Nursing

Jan Rose

It is Jan Rose's experience that the majority of those facilitating practice in occupational health nursing (OHN) are mentors whose role preparation varies considerably, with some having had no formal preparation for their teaching, learning, supervising and assessing role. We hope that despite the evident constraints and barriers to OHN specialist community practitioner education, those who are committed and determined to ensure that OHN education continues will be inspired by this chapter.

Introduction

Occupational health nursing is concerned with the protection and promotion of health and the prevention of ill health within the working environment. In order to achieve the aims of the specialist practitioner award – occupational health nursing, the student must develop a critical awareness of the political, social and economic influences that affect practice, and a deep understanding of hazards to health within the work environment and the changes in legislation related to the workplace. The work arena of occupational health nurses is dynamic and constantly changing for a multiplicity of reasons outside their control. Occupational health nurses must develop the ability to respond to pressures and demands placed upon them from more than one direction, as well as the ability to recognise and respond to the changing health needs of the workforce.

This chapter considers the challenges, difficulties and rewards inherent in supervising and assessing practice in industrial occupational health nursing settings. This focus on industry is deliberate as it is here that mentors will face the greatest challenges. A rationale and explanation of the strategies developed by the University of Wolverhampton is offered as one method of facilitating learning in a 'difficult to manage' specialism. Particular reference is made here to the theoretical framework outlined, based on a philosophy first espoused by Steinaker and Bell in 1979. This is not presented as a 'solution' to the teaching and learning problems common to occupational health nursing but as a base on which mentors can build strategies for facilitating the development of specialist practice that are appropriate to their specific occupational health setting.

Occupational health services

Occupational health services are defined in the International Labour Organization Convention 161 and Recommendation 171 (ILO 1985) which entrusts the occupational health service with essentially preventative functions to advise the employer, the workers and their representatives on:

- The requirements for establishing and maintaining a safe and healthy working environment to ensure optimal physical and mental health in relation to work
- The adaptation of work to the capabilities of workers in light of their state of physical and mental health.

The nature of OHN itself varies hugely and this has implications for the breadth of knowledge required of the specialist practitioner and, importantly, the ability of one mentor in one OHN setting to facilitate learning of a 'complete' specialist practitioner role. For instance, heavy engineering will require occupational health nurses to have knowledge of relevant statutes such as 'Permits to Work', whereas the food industry will require in-depth knowledge of food legislation, particularly in order to carry out pre-employment screening. Case study 4.4 in Chapter 4 demonstrates how the OHN mentor may need to utilise alternative practice placements and how the audit of practice will identify the educational potential of any one placement. Whether or not OHN fits well within specialist community practice is a matter for professional debate relating to the nature and current demands of the role. Although improving health at work through health promotion strategies is a main focus of the specialist practitioner role, informal discussion with OHNs suggests that their work is predominantly health and safety.

It is also important to note that OHN specialist students may remain in their existing employment area and be supported, at a distance, by a mentor working in a different practice. This is not ideal as it may limit the qualified practitioner's ability to facilitate learning and to support and assess specialist competencies, and it may limit the student's ability to experience a variety of OHN practices, with the possibility that the student completes the programme but with limited role development. However, with appropriate strategies (i.e. clinical supervision, see Chapter 6) suited to the student's individual learning needs it is possible for the mentor to facilitate learning 'at a distance' (Canham 1998).

Factors influencing the facilitation of learning in occupational health nursing

Supervision and assessment of practice in occupational health nursing education can be fraught with difficulties. Unlike other community specialist practices, such as health visiting, there is no mandatory requirement for nurses to hold the professional qualification before being employed in this specialist area. Occupational health nursing (OHN) differs from all other nursing disciplines, in that the majority of occupational health nurses are employed in the private sector (with the notable exception of occupational health for the NHS). In an industrial setting the primary focus is on the end product of that industry and employers perceive the occupational health nurse's role and value to the organisation as 'keeping the workers at work'. To the employer the function of the occupational health service is reducing sickness absence and thus improving productivity. To put it bluntly, to the employer, the industrial product is arguably of more importance than the employee and yet it is the employees who are the clients of the OHN. Occupational health nurses have to juggle their priorities between the client, the employer and in some cases, for example the food industry, the protection of the product. This conflict of interest creates one of the unique features of occupational health nursing.

The uniqueness of OHN affects specialist student practice in a number of ways. Whereas the philosophy of the nursing profession is to encourage learning of both students and colleagues, this can be constrained by the nature of employment of the OHN in industry. In most areas of specialist practice there are well established strategies for the provision of appropriate practice placements, even in areas where the qualification is not mandatory to practice (i.e. CMHN and GPN). In industry, employers may be reluctant to allow time for any type of educational input that is not related to, or likely to benefit, their own organisation. Employers may also not be willing to allow *their* occupational health nurses to spend time educating other nurses, who may be employed by someone else. Legally, occupational health nurses can only observe practice in other organisations. The employer is vicariously liable for the actions of his employees (Kloss 1994) and all non-crown employers have a duty to insure under the Employer's Liability (Compulsory Insurance) Act 1969 (Dimond 1990). If an OHN student is not an employee of that organisation then they are not covered by the employer's insurance and therefore cannot be allowed to practise.

'Having successfully completed my professional qualification, I was approached by my former tutor and asked if I could provide an alternative practice experience for a specialist student. Pleased to be asked and looking forward to the prospect of facilitating learning, I obtained permission for the specialist student to have a week's placement from my manager, the Personnel Director, and set up a full study programme. My manager was kept fully informed and approved of the programme I had arranged.

On the day in question, my manager was away at a meeting. It so happened that the Managing Director (whose head office was at another site) was visiting our site. When the occupational health student arrived at reception, the receptionist called to the telephonist to let me know that my visitor had arrived. The Managing Director (MD) overheard this comment. His immediate response was to inquire why the nurse was having visitors. My junior nurse appeared in my office and said that I was to go immediately to see the Production Director. When I arrived at his office I was asked why I was seeing visitors. I explained and said that I had been given permission to arrange this. The response was. "We don't pay you to teach students, the Managing Director wants your visitor off the site". I tried, in vain, to persuade the Production Director that this student had travelled a considerable distance to visit the company. In addition, far from being a casual visitor, my visitor was employed as an occupational health nurse in another industry and I pointed out that telling this colleague that they had to leave was impolite and reflected badly on the company. The response was "get your visitor off site now".

Case study 15.1 Denied access to learning

Case study 15.1 provides an extreme though graphic example of a traditional paternalistic management style (Handy 1993) and illustrates how occupational health nurses may find that they are restricted from becoming mentors by the nature of their employment. It is clear that some OHN employment acts against the furtherance of the specialism and that professional development is not the concern of the employer. The OHN may be able to develop working relationships with employers that enable mentoring to become a reality but this does need to be promoted in terms of the benefits to the company.

OHN university teachers realise that the availability of suitable placements depends on the goodwill of qualified occupational health professionals and their employers and the economic climate. As in all other specialist areas, practice needs to be audited for its ability to provide an appropriate learning environment and it is clear that within case study 15.1 any audit that took place was limited to the skills, knowledge and attributes of the mentor. In reality educational audit of OHN practice should include the employer's support of nurse education. It is worth noting that if an employer is willing in principle to support professional education, even the most paternalistic or rigid employment practices can be excellent learning opportunities for specialist students, providing critical, practical insight into the particular dynamics of the workplace. However, few employers will agree to having their OH service audited and this creates major difficulties for OHN practitioners in managing ENB requirements (Bamford & Warner 1998).

A more positive perspective

Fortunately for occupational health nurse education, many employers are understanding and helpful and often see the request to facilitate learning as a sign of the high quality of the occupational health service they provide.

One of the most positive comments frequently received from practitioners is that having students encourages them to critically evaluate their own area of practice. Contact with the HEI makes them aware of what is happening to occupational health at a national and international level and enables the development of OHN networks. The work arena of the occupational health nurse can vary considerably depending on the particular employing organisation. Occupational health nurses know the specific hazards and legislative requirements of their own organisation in considerable depth and yet can be unaware of the needs of other organisations. The cross-fertilisation of ideas exchanged with practitioners and specialist students from different settings provides a rich learning experience for both mentor and learner.

Although there may be many challenges to be faced, most occupational health nurses volunteer to become mentors because they gain considerable professional satisfaction from facilitating learning. The role of the mentor in OHN can be one that encourages debate regarding best practice, increases motivation and commitment to work for the OHN mentor, and can develop the company as a practice teaching exemplar.

Strategies for bridging the practice-theory gap in occupational health nursing

Prior to the introduction of specialist community practice, which included OHN (UKCC 1994), the occupational health programme at the University of Wolverhampton had developed a strategy for attempting to bridge the theory-practice gap. This was through a mentoring scheme in which an experienced and qualified occupational health nurse would mentor an OHN student (pre UKCC 1994). At that time, the OHN student was required to have practice placements in a number of OHN organisations over the period of the course. For these practice placements, objectives were set and an educational taxonomy was used to assess the student's progress (Nyatanga & Bamford 1990).

The range of ability and skills of specialist students entering OHN can be considerable. Since there is no mandatory requirement to have the professional qualification before being employed in this specialism, it is not uncommon for nurses to be in OH practice for up to ten years before they undertake specialist education. On the other hand full-time students may not be employed in OHN at all though may have considerable prior experience as post-registered practitioners. Because of this variation in students' learning needs, a grid based on Steinaker and Bell's (1979) experiential taxonomy (originally devised by Nyatanga *et al.* (1989) was developed to assess the extent of exposure, participation, identification, internalisation and dissemination (EPIID) occurring through each practical placement experience.

The grid consists of four columns (see Fig. 15.1). The first column contains the set objectives or competencies for the practical placement. The second column identifies the initial (present) level of mastery (ILOM). The third column is the expected level of mastery (ELOM) and the final column the actual (achieved) level of mastery (ALOM). Initial mastery identifies the student's existing skills in relation to specialist practice and thus establishes the time and level of student-mentor interaction necessary (Nyatanga & Bamford 1990). The expected level of mastery is established by the programme curriculum and in relation to specialist practice would be at dissemination in all

Placement objectives	ILOM					ELOM					ALOM				
	E	P	I	I	D	E	P	I	I	D	E	P	I	I	D
1.1 Critically analyse the role and function of the occupational health nurse															
1.2 Assess the environmental and safety risk factors in the organisation and provide a strategy for minimising risk															
1.3 Critically evaluate the principles of hazard control and justify the essential factors necessary for a major environmental disaster plan															
1.4 Critically evaluate self as OHN and identify potential in clinical nursing audit, contributing to research and supporting professional colleagues															
1.5 Critically analyse the impact of legislation on OH practice (relevance of statutes, guidance notes and Approved Codes of Practice)															

Fig. 15.1 Clinical nursing practice – application of ENB (1995) learning outcomes to the experiential taxonomy grid.

areas by the end of the course. Actual level of mastery is completed by the student and the mentor at the end of the learning experience.

To place this framework within the context of specialist practitioner preparation, one of the areas for development in occupational health nursing (ENB 1995) is:

Clinical nursing practice
● Assess, plan, provide and evaluate specialist clinical nursing care to meet nursing and occupational health needs

- Assess, manage and provide care in clinical emergencies, critical and environmental incidents to ensure care and safety
- Promote the appropriate and effective use of occupational health services in the workplace.

These specific learning outcomes can be incorporated into the experiential taxonomy (ET) grid, couched in terms of objectives or competencies to be achieved (see Fig. 15.1).

Helen White is a part-time specialist practitioner student who currently is employed as the sole nurse in OH by a food processing company. As a part-time student Helen uses her own work environment to meet specialist practice outcomes, whilst supported by a mentor working for a NHS Trust.

Helen meets with her mentor to identify where Helen feels that she is on the ET continuum, in terms of her existing knowledge and expertise. The mentor identifies that Helen is at the level of internalisation with regard to knowledge of relevant statutes and their application to the food industry (1.5 on Fig. 15.1). Helen is also able to transfer knowledge of health and safety legislation to areas relevant to the NHS with some ease.

Helen's own organisation does not have a major environmental disaster plan and although competent in knowledge of the legislation, Helen lacks confidence in advising senior management of the need for this (1.3 on Fig. 15.1). Helen feels quite happy advising employees on a one-to-one basis, but the thought of making a presentation or writing a report to the Managing Director creates anxiety. The mentor discusses with Helen the disaster plan formulated by the NHS occupational health service and enables Helen to formulate a plan for her own organisation and to prepare a report for senior management. Helen subsequently finds an improvement in confidence when approaching senior management on other issues.

As Helen progresses through the level of learning from exposure to an experience to its ultimate dissemination, so the mentor passes from being an advisor to an appraiser (Kenworthy & Nicklin 1989). During clinical supervision, the mentor assesses to what extent the learning experiences have influenced Helen's behaviour and uses the ET framework to identify the level that Helen has achieved.

Case study 15.2 Using an experiential taxonomy

Summary

This chapter has discussed some of the difficulties experienced by mentors in meeting the requirement for supervising and assessing practice within the field of occupational health nursing. Whether occupational health nursing fits comfortably into this unified model of specialist community practice is debatable. Due to legal restrictions on practice in other organisations it may not be feasible to allow mentors to supervise practice within the student's organisation if the two are different. The strategies developed at the University of Wolverhampton to address bridging the theory-practice gap using experiential taxonomy (Steinaker & Bell 1979) have been outlined and demonstrate that this particular taxonomy is appropriate to accommodate the considerable range of knowledge and experience of occupational health nurses.

Chapter 16

District Nursing

Anne Robinson

There can be no doubt that much of district nursing was rocked by the findings of the Audit Commission (1999), even though experienced practitioners knew that the profession desperately needed to move forward. With the aid of expert mentors, the next generation of district nurses will be very different practitioners from their predecessors. Anne Robinson identifies those areas of practice of great significance to a changing service; leadership, user lead and collaboration. This chapter also provides detail of how mentors can utilise management techniques (for example SWOT analyses) and reflection to promote learning through practice.

Introduction

District nurses deliver most of the professional care provided in patients' homes. It is a highly valued, respected, responsive service and an essential component in the complex pattern of support needed to sustain people at home. The demand for the service is rising and improvements within it are recognised as necessary to the modernisation of the NHS (DoH 1997a; Audit Commission 1999). The agenda for change aims to ensure the NHS makes best use of resources and delivers better, more responsive services. Systems and structures are to be established within the not too distant future to monitor the effectiveness of both performance and service provision (DoH 2000a). The changes envisaged will have a profound effect on the way district nursing services are managed, organised and delivered in the future, with the implications for the profession being onerous. It would be impossible to examine the role of the mentor within district nursing without exploring in more depth some of these factors that are impacting on the profession.

The aim of this chapter is to explore some of these challenges, identify the skills that future practitioners will require and discuss strategies that the mentor can utilise in promoting the development of these with district nursing students.

Policy context

Policy changes of the past decade have had enormous effect on the district nurse's role. Changes within organisational structures, skill mix, fundholding, community care and nurse prescribing have all influenced how roles have evolved and developed. It is apparent that further changes lie ahead (see Chapter 2). A recent review of district nursing highlighted the constraints and demands being placed on the service (Audit Commission 1999). For example, changing demographic and social trends have resulted in reductions in hospital stay, and increasing numbers of the elderly and patients with acute and chronic conditions are nursed at home with fewer families available to care for them. The likelihood that these trends will continue in the future has significant resource implications for district nurses.

The Audit Commission report also described a service that was demand-led and not well defined, with an imperfect referral process resulting in district nurses working under increasing pressure, juggling case-loads to manage workloads. It highlighted the need for case-load reviews and regular profiling as essential to improve the efficiency of the service, ensuring that resources are targeted at those with greatest need. A variation in the quality of the care that patients received was also apparent, with evidence that clinically effective care was not always introduced and outcomes were poorly evaluated.

The management role of the district nurse was also explored. The findings suggested a need for district nurses to delegate more clinical work to the team to provide more time for clinical leadership and management, which would have a direct impact on improving patient care. Trusts were provided with clear recommendations as to how the service could be modernised. These included:

- Clearer definitions of the role of the service, with improved referral processes
- Collaborative approaches with social services to ensure social care needs are met
- Tackling poor clinical performance through clinical audit and clinical supervision
- Regular audit and review of case-loads to ensure effective use of skills and resources
- Investment in the management and leadership roles of district nurses to enable them to fulfil their role in clinical and team management.

Implications for district nursing

The Audit Commission findings clearly indicate that many practices will need to change to meet the changing requirements of practice, which are based on the health needs of the local population (DoH 1999a).

Translating policy into the context of practice suggests a need for practitioners to be able to take managerial responsibility for the case-load and also function in a leadership role over and above that of team co-ordinator to ensure that:

- Opportunities for practice and service development are established through health needs assessment to meet local need

- Multi-disciplinary, inter-agency approaches to service development are established, using joint protocols, standards and guidelines to standardise care
- Resources are secured at an organisational level for service developments and to influence the commissioning process
- Case-loads, existing services and skill mix are critically reviewed to develop new patterns of working and ensure effective use of resources
- Training and educational needs of the team are established to support team development linked to needs of the PHCT and the organisation's business plans
- Clinical audit is utilised to evaluate effectiveness of services.

(Audit Commission 1999)

Challenges for the mentor

It is against this changing context of care that mentors face the challenge of preparing practitioners for their future role. It is evident that demands on the service will continue, but current patterns of delivery and organisation will need to be restructured to accommodate changes within the coming decade. The greatest impact will be on the role of qualified district nurses who will need to review current practice and their leadership and management role to meet the current modernisation programme. In case study 16.1 a nurse executive of a personal medical service (PMS) discusses the skills that will be imperative for future practitioners.

'There is a need for the district nurses to develop their leadership roles within the nursing team, across the PHCT and to be involved with developments within PCGs and PCTs. This is a huge agenda; they need to implement clinical governance at a local level, and lead practice development in line with the needs of the community. In future we will be looking for district nurses with evidence of a portfolio career who can clearly demonstrate that they have the ability to take the service forward and contribute to the development and implementation of strategy. You can see how in the future, this will be a consideration in the selection and appointment of staff...'

Case study 16.1 The need for practitioner development: views of a nurse executive (personal medical service)

Establishing leadership within primary care can be problematic. The context of primary care with its hierarchical structures and organisational overlaps creates particular challenges requiring practitioners who are able to challenge rigid patterns of team and organisational functioning (West & Poulton 1997a).

The most important quality in leadership is being able to challenge the existing status quo and getting other people to work together (Shuldham 1997). However, the professional culture within district nursing has been described as non-challenging, possibly creating barriers to change (Griffiths & Luker 1997). Challenging roles and responsibilities and implementing new approaches to service provision requires the leader to utilise constructive, empowering strategies to support and enable the team to move forward. Not only do mentors have to be willing to critically examine their own working practices but also those of other team members. This must be achieved in a constructive way to enable change to be implemented. Furthermore, support from the wider organisation and the PHCT is essential in achieving this.

The teaching and learning environment

The importance of preparing specialist practitioners with skills in critical thinking cannot be overstated. Promoting this level of thinking is challenging for both student and mentor (see Chapter 4). Observing a good role model can help students become critical thinkers; this requires that the mentor adopts this approach within practice and their mentoring role (Brookfield 1987). Critical thinking is fostered in an atmosphere where students can question and challenge practice. To promote the development of critical thinking, students need encouragement and support. Their progress has to be regularly evaluated. They need an environment where they feel safe, where they can be challenged but do not feel threatened, and where they are listened to and valued (Brookfield 1987). Central to the success of this being achieved therefore is the student-mentor relationship and an agreed learning contract negotiated at the onset of the learning programme (Brookfield 1987).

The starting point for the mentor is to identify the student's learning needs in relation to their practice competencies for specialist practice. This requires assessing the student's learning needs and developing a negotiated learning contract. This can provide the student with a clear focus for their learning and can facilitate the development of a programme pertinent to individual need. A learning contract provides students with an active role within their learning, with the clear responsibility for their learning outcomes (Quinn 1995).

Sarah had been accepted for sponsorship on the full-time course within an organisation that she had not been employed in previously. She was an experienced staff nurse who had worked within the community for four years as a D grade staff nurse. Her main responsibilities had been treatment room duties and delegated visits. Trust policies in her previous work had not allowed her to undertake first visits. During this time she had completed various academic courses and study days, she was very experienced in wound care and she had a good knowledge of palliative care. She had attended the PCG nursing meetings and was nurse representative on the clinical governance forum for her practice. She was also a school governor for several years and had been involved in policy development, recruitment and appointment of staff, and budgetary decisions.

Case study 16.2 A student profile

The student who has worked within the community setting as a staff nurse will have different needs from a student who is a direct entrant with little or no community experience. Various strategies have been described in previous chapters to assess students' learning needs to enable mentors to develop a learning contract and programme pertinent to each student's requirement. The one I have found useful is a SWOT analysis (Fig. 16.1).

Strengths: e.g.
- Specific clinical skills
- Personal qualities
- Experience in primary care
- Formal education
- Qualifications

Weaknesses (areas for development): e.g.
- Knowledge of primary care
- Specific clinical skills
- Policies, guidelines, protocols
- Networks
- Referral systems
- Assessment skills
- Team working
- Management skills
- Time management

Opportunities (for learning): e.g.
- Shadowing
- Critical discussions
- Case studies
- Reflection
- Critical incidents
- Clinical nurse specialists
- Placement visits

Threats (barriers to overcome to ensure learning opportunities are maximised) e.g.
- Time for discussion, debate and reflection
- Skills in reflection
- Relationship between mentor and student

Fig. 16.1 SWOT analysis.

This process can enable both student and mentor to identify the student's strengths and areas for development, which will be addressed within the learning programme. Opportunities for learning can be identified and barriers, which may detract from this happening, can be addressed.

The list provided in Fig. 16.1 is not intended to be prescriptive but merely to provide a framework to support the development of the learning contract.

An assessment of her learning needs helped Maggie (Sarah's mentor) to identify Sarah's strengths and identify the areas she needed to develop. Maggie was then able to develop a programme pertinent to Sarah's needs, in relation to the care management and clinical leadership competencies.

Patients were selected from the case-load to provide Sarah with the appropriate experiences she needed to help develop the skills and knowledge. Maggie used her knowledge of the organisation to identify appropriate placement visits. Opportunities for joint visits were agreed as well as time for discussions related to her experiences.

Time is frequently identified as the greatest problem for both the student and the mentor. The need for quality dedicated time for critical discussion, debate and reflection on practice is seen as essential for learning in practice (see Chapter 5). Mentors who promote this approach to learning and encourage lateral thinking are highly respected and valued by their students. However, it is apparent from discussions with students that these strategies are not always utilised or adopted. The contract provides an opportunity to negotiate the time needed to achieve this, ensuring that both students' and mentors' needs and expectations are met.

Sarah was encouraged to keep a reflective diary and to document her learning from practice. These were later used as a basis for the discussions between herself and Maggie. Sarah was able to identify issues in practice that she needed to explore and Maggie was then able to facilitate the process by helping her reflect on practice. By exploring the evidence base to practice she was able to discuss her findings with Maggie. Opportunities for service development were discussed, implications of the nursing team, PHCT and the organisation were identified and barriers that would need to be overcome were explored.

From these discussions Sarah was able to gain a greater understanding of the leadership role and insight into the complexities of implementing change within primary care and the nursing team. She was able to draw on her theoretical knowledge and discuss its relevance within the context of practice. Maggie and Sarah were then able to identify further learning opportunities to meet learning needs identified from undertaking this approach.

Reflection is recognised as a strategy to enable learning from practice (Benner 1984) (see Chapter 5). Schön (1987) suggests that by using reflective processes practitioners can stand back from practice, identify the problem-solving process used and gain insight into professional knowledge. Reflection presents an opportunity for nurses to revisit their existing practice (Driscoll 1994), illuminating the knowledge used enabling them to share their expertise (Ford & Walsh 1994). This leads to improvements in practice by providing the professional with alternative ways of seeing problems that cannot be dealt with in books (Driscoll 1994).

Reflection also provides an opportunity for mentors, who are working at the interface of change, to be able to articulate the knowledge utilised in practice, uncovering practice-based knowledge (see Chapter 5). By adopting an approach which includes problem-based learning and reflection, students are encouraged to adopt a more critical, analytical approach to practice, promoting the development of both critical and lateral thinking. The critical discussion between student and mentor provides an opportunity for the student to clearly demonstrate the integration of theory and practice.

The mentor's role is to facilitate the process, challenge the student appropriately and assess the student's competency in practice. Evidence presented by the student can be utilised within the practice portfolio, demonstrating a rationale for practice based on evidence-based practice.

Conclusion

Policy documents are indicating that roles will have to change drastically to ensure that services are developed to meet the clinical governance agenda. How this agenda will unfold is unclear. The implications of major organisational change and the full impact of policy change have yet to be realised. It is quite apparent that district nurses are central to policies being implemented locally and will have a key role in taking primary care forward. It is imperative that they have the skills to cope with this challenging agenda and the ability to influence the development of the profession and community services.

Chapter 17

School Nursing

Jennie Humphries

This chapter on mentoring in school nursing (school health) is very welcome as it was not that many years ago that the practice of school nursing was taught by health visitors. Jennie Humphries' experiences in both practice and education and her commitment to the development of school nursing enable her to examine the issues that confront the mentor and provide promising solutions.

Introduction

Education for nurses to become school nurses is not mandatory, though the call to make it so has been made for several years (Abraham 1990; Sadler 1991; CPHVA 2000a). However, from 1998 school nurse education gained equal status with other specialist community practitioner courses. This recognition is endorsing that the standard and quality of education and training must be the same for nurses who work with children of school age and represents a vital step in acknowledging the expertise of school nurses.

The role of the school nurse specialist practitioner

School nursing practice is changing rapidly. There is a shift from screening and surveillance of healthy individuals towards selectivity and promoting the health of whole school populations. The framework for school nursing suggested by DeBell & Jackson (2000) encapsulates the recommendations of *Making a Difference* (DoH 1999a) and *Saving Lives: Our Healthier Nation* (DoH 1999b), advocating a public health approach to the role. Whilst this has been the focus of specialist community practitioner (SCP) courses, as outlined by the UKCC (1994), the reality of school nursing practice has often been very different. A diversity of practice can be useful in addressing local variations and needs but the ad hoc nature of service development has meant that an uneven service is provided and quality initiatives are often not disseminated. There continue to be parts of the UK that adopt a medical model approach to school nursing with the service essentially being led by community medical officers (CMOs) and nurses functioning as hand maidens at school medicals (Ottewill & Wall 1990). Even those that have abandoned this format may still offer a production line screening and surveillance service leaving school nurse practitioners with little time to develop the role to better meet the needs of contemporary school-aged children and young people (Clarke 2000; Humphries & Tonge 2000). Conversely the CPHVA (1998) describes a range of health promoting activities and interventions that school nurses are engaged in, both with whole school populations and in one-to-one interventions.

This variety presents the mentor for school nurses with a challenge in ensuring that the student receives a quality of learning that reflects the potential, and the actual, nature of the specialist practitioner. Clearly if a job specification states that school nurses should be able to measure and weigh children and undertake hearing and vision screening, this has to be included in the training. If school nursing is to move forward, however, other characteristics of specialist practitioner functions have to be addressed. The national framework (CPHVA 1999, 2000a; DeBell & Jackson 2000) identifies four areas of practice for school nurses:

- Healthy lifestyles
- Mental health
- Children with chronic and complex health needs
- Vulnerable children – 'looked after' children and others experiencing social exclusion, which includes particular groups such as refugees, excluded school children and victims of violence.

Significantly the national framework refers to the education that school nurses require in meeting the needs of the client group. It also acknowledges that understanding the roles and responsibilities of others is essential to the development of effective collaborative working needed to meet the complexity of health needs of school age children and young people.

Mentor preparation

The role of the mentor involves commitment to the student and their learning. A fundamental requirement is a desire to do the job. School nurses with the high levels of motivation and dedication to professional development that are essential prerequisites in a mentor are unsurprisingly often the people who volunteer for the role. There are others who may fail initially to recognise their own capabilities or suitability for the job but have it acknowledged by their manager or peers and gladly agree to be a mentor when asked.

Karen qualified as a school nurse five years ago. She is well respected by her peers and has led several initiatives developing school nursing. Last year Karen undertook the ENB teaching and assessing course and enjoys having student nurses on placement. Karen is confident in her abilities to be a mentor but is concerned about how the responsibility will impinge on her current role.

Karen is right to be concerned. She has a busy workload and recognises that her own professional competence cannot be compromised. Karen's manager Bobbie agrees that some of the money earmarked for covering the student's case-load can be used to reduce Karen's case-load.

Other mechanisms that can be used:

- If it is acceptable to the mentor it may be possible to negotiate an increase in hours for the period of time the student is with her
- Sharing some of the mentor's existing workload between colleagues
- As the student progresses she will be given increasing responsibility and passing a school to the student for her own practice development will ease the burden later in the course
- Putting new initiatives on hold for the duration of the course or bringing in other team members and later the student to assist.

Case study 17.1 Managing mentorship and existing role commitments

Mentor support

To competently fulfil the role of mentor dedicated time is required and thus the current workload has to be assessed and should be adjusted to reflect the additional responsibilities (CPHVA 2000b). A significant source of support will be from the manager and, if there is one, the practice educator. Support from colleagues on both a practical and psychological level should be welcomed. Support groups of mentors from the different community specialties can be helpful in allowing examination of specific and general issues relating to student learning within a locality.

Clearly collaboration with the HEI is an essential part of the specialist practitioner programme and support for the mentor is part of this. Preparation days for all mentors from the different community specialties allow cross-fertilisation of ideas and sharing of experiences and concerns. Support meetings organised at regular intervals usually include a mixture of group meetings at the HEI and visits by the university to student placements. It is important that the mentor has a means of accessing a named university teacher between times should any situation arise for which they are unprepared and need guidance.

Although recommendations from the CPHVA (2000b, p.5) are that, 'All community practitioners responsible for the practice education of specialist community practitioner students must hold a recordable teaching qualification on the UKCC register', they acknowledge that this is not the present situation. They do urge that this should be reviewed locally and nationally. School nurse mentors will find that undertaking mentor preparation will provide support and encourage the development of skills to assist in teaching, facilitating and assessing. Depending on the format of the course, the mentor will have access to peer and academic support. It may be that the mentor's own experience of being a learner allows an empathic rapport with the school nurse student.

Louise is currently undertaking mentor preparation at a local HEI. As part of the programme she has to progress through various learning opportunities and one of these involves providing Pam, her student, with feedback about a health education session. Louise is to be assessed on this procedure. It is important that Pam is cognisant of the procedure involved and that she gives informed consent as being observed can add to the stresses that students frequently experience during such an intensive learning programme. However Louise is also a student and has her own learning needs so hopefully Pam will empathise and agree to participate in strategies that allow Louise to learn also.

Case study 17.2 Being a mentor and a 'student'

Fostering a positive student-mentor relationship

School nurse students enter the course with a range of skills and experiences. Some may have years of experience as a school nurse, whilst others may be new to the role and perhaps to community nursing. This variety enhances the learning in the classroom as students share their expertise. However, the needs of these students are different and the skills of the mentor are vital in ensuring that, whatever the background of the student, the learning in practice complements this. It is necessary for the mentor to harness previous expertise; this helps the student to realise that prior experiences are important and is a tangible recognition that the mentor acknowledges the learner's existing qualities. For some learners the prospect of becoming a student after perhaps years of high-level expertise in their previous role can be daunting and the mentor must bear in mind that the nurse may feel vulnerable because of the new status as student.

Vicki had come onto the school nursing course without any experience of the role. Her mentor, Linda, was sensitive to this and was initially guided by Vicki's own learning needs. During the first semester Vicki gained experience by observing Linda and others but seemed reluctant to participate in practice alone. Linda did not force the issue but gently encouraged Vicki to take on more responsibility with Linda nearby. For example, during Year 7 health interviews Linda arranged to stay on the school premises so that Vicki knew assistance and advice was available if she needed it. This increased Vicki's confidence so that she was later able to take the school as the named school nurse for the final semester of the course.

Case study 17.3 Enabling student self confidence

Facilitating the achievement of learning outcomes

One academic year is a relatively short time for the student to gain the knowledge and skills to become a school nurse, and a significant task for the mentor is to ensure that student experience in practice reflects the student's needs in relation to the learning outcomes. The learning outcomes for the course will be clearly documented so that the student, mentor and university teacher are all working towards the same goals.

Degree level students are expected to take considerable responsibility for their own learning; guidance and facilitation are the essential elements of the mentor role in the process. By empowering students in this way they are able to acknowledge the learning experience as individuals and recognise that not everyone learns in the same way or at the same pace (*Nursing Times Learning Curve* 1999).

Vicki and her mentor Linda felt comfortable with the learning process. Some of the learning objectives were not being achieved as rapidly as for other students on the course but both were confident that they would be in time for the summative assessment. The university teacher was kept informed of progress and was satisfied with Vicki's progression in both theory and practice. However, Chris, the school nurse manager, was concerned with what she perceived as Vicki's slow progress and worried that Vicki would not be able to function as a school nurse on qualifying. Previous students had been working as unqualified school nurses for some time before undertaking the school nurse course and Chris began to question her own decision to employ Vicki. Chris was passing her anxieties to Vicki and Linda causing them to doubt their ability as student and mentor. The university teacher at the HEI was able to allow all three to explore the issues by arranging a joint meeting. Vicki and Linda were reassured that their management of learning was entirely appropriate and many of Chris' concerns were assuaged. On completion of the course Vicki achieved all the learning outcomes and is now practising as a competent, effective school nurse. With the benefit of hindsight Chris can see that Vicki's preparation for the role was right for her and hopefully will feel confident in employing others without prior school nursing experience.

Case study 17.4 Am I doing it right? Using a tripartite relationship

Students on the course must work towards achieving the theoretical and the practice learning outcomes and significantly they must function to ensure that integration of the two elements is achieved. Mentors are not expected to assess the student's academic abilities but students have to be able to demonstrate that their practice is underpinned by relevant theories. Reflecting on learning and practice will assist both student and mentor in this procedure. By utilising various mechanisms in the learning process the mentor can facilitate reflection-on-action (Schön 1987). One of the most useful methods for encouraging this is during one-to-one discussion, allowing the student to explore rationales for practice, analyse reading and classroom learning and stimulate critical debate. Gillings and Davies (1998) emphasise the necessity for a regular time commitment for such reflection. Formulating aims and objectives for the meeting concentrates both student and mentor on the task.

Clearly the school nurse mentor requires a sound knowledge base and skills in stimulating the thought processes of the student. These include skills and knowledge of the reflective process (Barry 1999) as well as expertise in school nursing. Possible areas for exploration will arise throughout the student's learning, for example:

- A student experience in practice whether working alone or with others
- An observation experience including that of the mentor, other health care professionals and the range of others who work with children and young people
- Student's reading or classroom experience
- Student's assignments, which are designed to develop the learner's skills in theory-practice integration.

Assessment

One of the functions of the mentor is to monitor the performance of the student to ensure that they are safe and competent practitioners capable of delivering safe and effective service to the public. Maintaining standards is a cornerstone of *A First Class Service* (DoH 1998a); there is a major focus on quality and effective monitoring of care, so clearly the mentor has to be confident that the student achieves the learning outcomes.

The nature of the specialist school nurse practitioner is such that competence is required in working with individuals, with families and within the public health domain, for example in working with whole schools and with school age children in the wider community. The mentor has to ensure that students have access to a range of school nursing activity and are able to develop this expertise. Importantly, as specialist community practitioners school nurses must learn to function in a way that addresses the needs of contemporary practice.

Gillings and Davies (1998) emphasise that the evaluation of student performance is a continuous process. They note that regular meetings allow for careful examination of learning outcomes and the development of a realistic and achievable action plan for the student's future development.

The ultimate responsibility for assessment of practice lies with the mentor but the academic staff should be consulted if problems arise in practice that cannot be resolved between student and mentor.

Strategies for student support

The support from the mentor to the student during the course is essential. Issues that arise are varied and include providing advice and guidance in respect of course theory, the practical elements of school nursing and the relationship between the two. In addition the mentor will be exposed to problems that the student is experiencing relating to learning and perhaps in her personal life (Jarvis & Gibson 1997). Marson (1990) advocates that being an effective facilitator of learning requires the qualities of good nursing: empathy, sensitivity and the ability to respond in an appropriate way. Just as nurses should acknowledge their own competence and seek help from others when necessary, mentors must recognise their own limitations and be aware of other systems that can be of benefit to students.

Anne began to feel very stressed in the second semester of the course. She was experiencing changes in her personal life and had developed some minor health problems. At first she told no one about her difficulties and presented a brave front to the academic staff and to Jean, her mentor. An incident during practice served as the catalyst when Jean tried to explore why Anne had made an uncharacteristic mistake during a routine session. No harm was done and Jean was not being critical but Anne became distressed and her personal and academic difficulties surfaced. Jean was supportive to Anne but she herself felt overwhelmed and at a loss as to how to deal with the problems. Fortunately both Jean and Anne recognised that the situation could not be dealt with without other help. The academic staff made arrangements for Anne to attend the student counselling service, and devised an assignment submission programme giving Anne later submission dates. Anne did not qualify with her peers but did successfully complete the course four weeks later. Jean's perception in distinguishing between normal stress often experienced by students and that requiring additional help was certainly instrumental in Anne becoming a school nurse.

Case study 17.5 Facilitating appropriate student support

Conclusion

Perhaps more than any other area of specialist community nursing practice the role of the school nurse is developing at a remarkable pace with a shift of focus that enables school nurses to be the professional leaders within school health services and significant contributors to the public health agenda for the school-age population (DeBell & Jackson 2000). This places responsibility on newly qualified practitioners to put their skills and knowledge into action so that the impetus is maintained to assist with this exciting period of school nursing practice. They cannot do this without high quality education, half of which is facilitated by mentors. This chapter has discussed some of the issues in relation to this with respect to being a mentor in the field of school nursing. Hopefully it will prove beneficial to those who undertake this challenging but enjoyable and rewarding role.

Chapter 18

Being a Specialist Practitioner Student

Carole Wills

This chapter is a brief account of Carole Wills' experience of undertaking a specialist practitioner course (health visiting), and includes personal reflections of her experiences during the course, the realities of practice on completing the course and the subsequent development of her role as a mentor.

Introduction

I commenced the specialist practitioner course following 12 years' experience of working within the acute and community sectors. In the community I had worked as a registered nurse within a district nurse 'bank' and then later as a practice nurse. A year prior to commencing the course I secured a part-time post working as a community staff nurse for a local NHS Trust, within a health visiting team, alongside my practice nurse post. This was a planned move in an effort to enhance my application for sponsorship for the course rather than applying for sponsorship as an external applicant.

I opted for the part-time route of the BSc (Hons) Community Specialist Practitioner Award and the ENB Higher Award for a number of reasons, the most important of which was that, as a mother, I had to consider the impact on my family life of working and studying full time. I therefore assumed that the part-time mode would be less pressured and thus not affect my family life too greatly.

The practicalities of becoming a part-time student

The programme was split into modules of study and consisted of 50% practice and 50% theory. This involved one day a week in university and one day a week in the practice placement. I was to continue my work as a community staff nurse as well as my two days of study, totalling 3.5 days of 'working' time, but would have to leave my post as a practice nurse. This meant I had to drop to a basic staff nurse grade for the duration of the course. I thus continued to work as a practice nurse on a relief basis when time allowed, both for financial reasons and in order to retain my clinical skills. I believed that this would facilitate a wider scope of employment on completion of the course should there be no health visiting opportunities. It also meant, however, that I was often working almost full time, which I had wanted to avoid.

I later discovered that the full time mode included two days' attendance at university, two days within the practice placement and one day study leave. As a part-time student I did not receive any study leave and this inequality did serve to cause initial frustrations with most of my part-time counterparts as the stresses of part-time study combined with another job role became evident.

Practice placement

My practice placement was to be within the rural practice where I worked as a staff nurse. This meant that the health visitor I worked with would also be my mentor. The health visitor had not undertaken the mentor role for many years and was concerned about her ability to facilitate this role. It is acknowledged that mentors will require preparation for this role (Oldman 1999), support from the educational establishment (Jackson 1994) and some will need the opportunity to study at level III (Hudson and Forester 1995). My mentor identified her needs and enquired about updating her mentor qualification. She found that she did not have enough CATs (credit accumulation points) to access the university programme unless she underwent formal accreditation of prior learning (APL) assessment or accreditation of experiential learning (APEL), which she did not wish to undertake.

I had no doubt about her ability to facilitate my practical experience but there were times when I felt that we would both have benefited from her having updated on current educational issues and methods in more depth, e.g. reflective practice and critical analysis. It might also have lessened her anxieties about facilitating the development of a student at degree level. I felt the university teacher helped in this respect essentially by encouraging us to explore different kinds of knowledge and develop further understanding of how practice-based and experiential knowledge integrated within theoretical frameworks. This reinforced the fact that different types of knowledge inform each other, so my mentor's knowledge and experience were valued in the same way as the theoretical knowledge used to guide much of the programme.

Reflecting on the student role

From my own perspective, I did not anticipate the feelings of frustration which accompanied my reversion to a 'student' and to the narrow confines of my staff nurse role. I felt I had lost the autonomy, responsibilities and expertise that my previous practice nurse role had provided. I had been acknowledged as an 'expert' within this role and now was merely a 'student' who also worked as a staff nurse. On reflection I believe I was probably experiencing the loss of what Benner (1984) describes as 'expert status' and was floundering within the novice to competent stages of entering a new profession and developing my health visiting experience.

This frustration increased as the course progressed. My increasing skills, confidence, knowledge base and perception of holistic health required more than the routine activities for which I had been initially employed and I found my role becoming tedious. I found it frustrating to adhere to my staff nurse job description one day and then undertake more in-depth health visitor-related activities the next. In practice my mentor and I would often swap around visits and activities to facilitate my learning. In retrospect I was fortunate in the quantity and quality of the experiences I was able to undertake due to the flexibility of my staff nurse role. Had I not had the same health visitor who was my work colleague/manager as well as my mentor, I believe my experiences may have been very different. Other students had little flexibility to alternate practice days and thus were confined to the issues/practice events of that day.

Other positive aspects included studying within an environment where I was already an accepted member of the primary health care team and I already understood the roles and responsibilities of everyone working within the team. I also had knowledge of the 'system' and local community that brought benefits in patient knowledge and skills development as well as a knowledge basis of practice policies and procedures. Many of my student counterparts were working within their 'job' for three days a week (many within the acute sector, e.g. coronary care) and then in their practice placement for one day and university the other. Peer discussions during student breaks revealed feelings of isolation and a lack of understanding of the basics of health visiting. Many were undertaking the course with no post-registration community experience let alone health visiting. Oldman (1999) confirms this, stating that health visiting students are unlikely to have gained such experience, so I believe my situation must have been unusual in this respect. Many students began seeking community staff nursing posts within health visiting teams after the first few months, to offer extra support and insight. These posts, however, were very few but those who succeeded said that they felt more at ease with their skill development and were able to concentrate their efforts on learning about health visiting practice instead of 'swapping role hats' depending on the day of the week. This raises the need to increase the number of posts and opportunities which provide experience of working with health visitors.

University experience

The study day at university (Fridays) was split in two. The morning study consisted of core modules which all community disciplines studied together. I believe this environment paved the way for greater understanding and sharing of the experiences and roles of other disciplines, especially for those with no previous community experience. The afternoon sessions focused on specialist practice and all community groups separated to work within their specialist areas. It was felt within the health visiting group that much more time could have been devoted to health visiting practice and theory. This would, however, have implications for the length and content of the course, points which are currently being debated at a national level.

Home life

I did not want my study to impact too greatly on my family life and thus study was exclusively undertaken late in the evening, once my child was asleep. I developed a timetable for studying which kept weekends free for family activities and a couple of evenings with my partner and friends. This required great discipline and a pragmatic approach but I recognised that although I wanted to achieve a high quality degree I did not want to achieve it to the detriment of my family.

Despite having a supportive partner, the bulk of the household chores were mostly left to me and at times I did struggle to meet the demands of my family, work and study. The stresses associated with multiple role juggling are identified within the literature (Beck & Scrivastava, 1991), particularly when study is on a part-time basis and combined with childcare. I found this to be true, because during the two years of the course my daughter underwent two operations as well as suffering from ear infections, tonsillitis, chickenpox and scarlet fever! This placed a great deal of pressure on me and in order to cope required that my partner and I rearrange holidays and working schedules, and family helped out where possible. At times study became the lowest priority. Without the flexibility and understanding of my mentor, who allowed me to rearrange appointments and swap around working days, I do not know how I would have coped. This support was essential to my continuing with the course when times were difficult. However I believe that this flexibility was only possible because I worked in the same practice as a student and as a staff nurse.

The ENB Higher Award

One of the most challenging, yet beneficial areas of the course centred on the ENB Higher Award (ENB1991). McHale's small evaluative study (1998) suggests that practitioners who have undertaken the Higher Award use reflective practice to continually evaluate and update their practice and are more confident. The use of reflection has been much debated (positively and negatively) within the literature. I, however, have been able to incorporate this technique into my everyday practice and believe it to be a useful learning tool.

The Higher Award requires that practitioners demonstrate their ability to integrate ten key characteristics into their practice based on an identified need within the practice area. This involved identifying a practice issue which required change in some way, or a service innovation, and implementing and evaluating this change/innovation. The theoretical aspects were relatively straightforward – undertaking a literature search of the chosen area and identifying themes which would guide the innovation alongside the theories of change management, research, quality of care, resource management and teamwork etc. Tripartite agreements and meetings of the university teacher, the mentor and the student were used to guide the innovation. The mentor and myself relied heavily on the university teacher to disentangle the occasional web of confusion and guide us through Higher Award issues.

The practical issues were more complicated. The change implemented had to be continued once the student had left the practice placement and thus the change or innovation had to be something that was needed and would fit within the mentor's time allowance and ethos. As a health visiting student it was difficult to identify an area of practice which could be changed, owing to my limited experience of health visiting. I was also aware of the potential 'threat' that change posed to the mentor. It was of unspoken importance that the identified area did not criticise any aspect of personal practice. Although I eventually settled for an idea that did not inspire me totally, I learned a great deal. What became evident was that the process itself is a learning experience, and can be used in any situation where change is to be undertaken. I believe that this process facilitates the 'doing' side of reflective practice. Even in its simplest form, reflecting on practice may enable the practitioner to identify areas where change is needed. The Higher Award process then informs the practitioner of the next steps to facilitate that change. I have successfully utilised this process on several occasions since completing the programme to help bring about small changes within my practice area.

Consolidated practice?

The final part of the programme required all disciplines to work full time for a period of eight weeks in order to consolidate their practice. The mentor would allocate a small case-load of families with varying needs and would also be a source of support. My mentor felt strongly that this length of time was inadequate as with the previous traditional course much longer had been required. This may be true for traditional students or those with little community experience relying totally on the course practice component for their experience. However, this was not my belief or that expressed by fellow students during our many discussions. I felt that I had the advantage of having some health visiting and other community experience. I was not starting from the same point as other students and thus perhaps had developed competence at an earlier stage. I also believe that undertaking the course over two years allowed time for reflection and consolidation along the way, in comparison to some of the full-time students who fit the same amount of theoretical and practice learning into nine months, albeit the same amount of theory and practice days. I considered that degree level study had developed my critical/analytical skills as well as leadership skills to the point that I felt I was 'marking time'. I saw very little of my mentor during this consolidated practice component so perhaps her views were based more on being used to traditional methods of acquiring competence rather than concerns about my own personal competence. I felt more than ready to move on to a health visiting role.

On completing the course, whispers of possible vacancies but no concrete offers encouraged me to seek and secure a part-time health visiting post within a neighbouring NHS Trust. Other specialisms experienced the same plight. It seems wasteful and short-sighted that some Trusts should sponsor placements for specialist practitioner courses and yet not offer suitable posts to these successful students. I believe this raises issues regarding the current nature of workforce planning within the NHS.

Back to reality

The course had prepared me for many areas of practice which included the need to approach the role in a systematic way through undertaking a health needs assessment of the population and identifying priority areas based on this; but I was unprepared for staff sickness, maternity leave and the general lack of written data and knowledge about families, practice and the community with whom I would be working.

The six months of being a neophyte health visitor was the most stressful time I have ever experienced. It reinforced the need for preceptorship which in this particular area, was non-existent. Had it not been for the skills acquired in life-long learning, reflection, time management and priority setting through the course and previous experience, I do not know how I would have coped. I quickly learned child protection policies and further developed my skills in report writing and managing my priorities. I worked many more hours than I was paid for and had to take work home to ensure completion. In retrospect I cannot decide whether my experience was stressful because I was newly qualified or whether any other unsupported health professional in the same environment would have struggled in the same way. However, I believe that planned preceptor support would have reduced my feelings of isolation and would have offered practical support during a very stressful period.

Supporting other specialist practitioners

Since qualifying, my role has continued to evolve to take account of local and practice needs. I have developed my autonomous clinical assessment skills to facilitate minor illness clinics. I have also developed my teaching role which includes the induction and support of newly appointed community staff, updating experienced staff and supporting and facilitating learning for an experienced practice nurse undertaking the specialist practitioner programme.

I did have initial concerns about undertaking the role of mentor for a practice nurse because I did not have a mentor qualification and therefore questioned my own knowledge, skills and credibility in this area. My experience, however, is that these concerns were unfounded. I have utilised my experience and knowledge of practice nursing (an area where I had many years' experience), the specialist practitioner course (which I had recently completed) and current learning methods to facilitate our discussions of practice and theoretical issues. Building on my own experiences of working in general practice nursing and reflecting on my needs as a specialist practitioner student, we developed a relationship based on the need for support and guidance in key areas such as the integration of theoretical and practice issues and the ENB Higher Award process. The practice nurse and myself viewed our relationship as a partnership. We set aside protected time each week when we worked together to discuss and debate theory and practice issues, and how these in turn related to the current and future role of the practice nurse. These issues included policy changes, new clinical guidelines, quality audits and critical incidents etc.

I consider that it is the quality of the support which is of importance and not the fact of whether the supervisor is a mentor or currently belongs to that discipline. I believe the mentor should ideally emanate a quiet confidence, be approachable, flexible to the needs of the student, and above all ensure that time together is protected and valued. Some sessions may seem as though things are not moving forward but by spending time actively listening, critically analysing and reflecting upon situations, the way ahead often becomes clearer.

Conclusion

My experience of being a specialist practitioner student was rich and varied. At times I struggled to combine all of the course requirements with family life and work. This was made worthwhile by the sense of achievement experienced on completing assignments and achieving respectable marks. Overall, I have found higher education to be an unsettling yet inspiring experience. Unsettling in that I find I am continuously critically exploring areas of practice and identifying flaws which were not obvious to me previously; some I can do something about, others perhaps not. Inspiring in that I have now developed the knowledge and ability to critically analyse practice situations and change practice, and moreover I have confidence in my ability to do so. I am acutely aware of the needs of my fellow learners and colleagues and aim to support them to achieve their potential. Through the process of learning I have grown and developed personally as well as professionally. My knowledge of policy context and local need and my ability to reflect in and on practice means that I am one step ahead and intend to remain so. I no longer wait for others to voice the need for change and then instigate it; I can do it myself.

Chapter 19

Being a Mentor

Marjorie Cavanagh

We are indebted to Marjorie Cavanagh for using her personal time to write about her experiences as a mentor. There is no one better to tell the tale than someone who has the scars to prove it. Marjorie's approach to providing the best possible learning environment and opportunities for learning starts before the student has set foot in practice. For specialist students some of the strategies described here, for example clinical support groups, continue after qualification.

Introduction

My life as a district nurse and community practice teacher (now mentor) has been varied in both the type of student I have supported and in the degree of pleasure afforded by the experience. Specialist practitioner (district nurse) students invariably provide me with the greatest pleasures and challenges; individual students have contributed in many ways to the development of my own practice.

Each student comes to practice with specific and unique learning needs. I believe that the first days and weeks of the student placement are about exploring the person, finding out about each other, *knowing* the student (Rowntree 1987), discovering her/his needs and beginning to develop a special relationship within which optimum learning can be achieved. It is important that the mentor works alongside the student in order to discover individual learning needs and that, as a team, learning options and priorities are considered. Although some will come with a clear vision of their learning needs, others will need much more support and so the mentor will need to be alert and responsive in order to enable the student to reach her/his destination.

In this chapter I hope to be able to explicate the joys, pains and slight discomforts of being a mentor and provide some (mainly) experiential strategies for managing the practice learning process. I would not expect all mentors to follow my suit, as our practices are uniquely different, but I do hope that my experiences provide an insight into the reality of a complex role.

I present some dilemmas which are often impossible to solve alone and in starting off suggest that all mentors establish a strategy for educational support. This will always include colleagues in the higher education institute

(HEI) but should also include other local mentors (whatever specialism) and, of course, clinical supervision.

The learning environment

I work in a busy and often noisy (practice base) environment and am very much aware that the atmosphere in which students learn can be fundamental to their learning enjoyment and thus their relationship with life-long learning. The entirety of the learning environment is far more significant to students than the simple bricks and mortar (appearance and situation) of the building. For example, although students always need a quiet area where they are able to reflect and develop strategies for action, this can be less important than dedicated support from a committed mentor and the practice team.

Team approach to learning

For district nurse (and other specialist practice) students the transition to specialist practitioner includes learning how to be a team-member, while at the same time developing a clinical leadership role. Although the mentor is responsible for providing an appropriate learning environment within which to achieve this transition, it is vital that the team embraces an understanding of student need as well as an ownership of responsibility for student-support. The environment needs to be rich and stimulating and one in which practitioners respect each other. Students will thrive and grow if the atmosphere is caring and empathetic, where the student 'belongs' and where needs are respected (Rogers 1969).

To achieve this supportive environment, I always meet with the district nurse (DN) team before the student arrives, to explain the specialist student's learning outcomes in relation to the future role, clarifying that the student may be new to DN practice but will quickly have to assume both a team membership and a leadership role. Although there is much anecdote that suggests existing teams will act against specialist students achieving their learning outcomes, my experience is that with appropriate and timely introduction to the student, the team will actively encourage student achievement and indeed relish the opportunity to take part in learning activities. Team meetings and team supervision are useful for both the student and the team as they provide a forum for discussion of ideas and development of innovations in practice.

The student's introduction to practice

The first weeks of the practice placement are vital; during this time opportunities are sought for the learning environment to be enriched and introductions are made to other health care professionals and members of the wider primary care team. Networking is introduced as a measure in the development of infrastructures for appropriate care. The need for effective communication cannot be over-emphasised. I feel it is particularly important that the specialist student is introduced to both the primary care team and to patients as 'a qualified nurse who is undertaking a degree course in district nursing'. Without this rider, inappropriate relationships might develop, based more on the perception of 'student' than developing specialist practitioner.

Identifying learning needs and opportunities for learning

Students need to have some idea of their own learning needs – a starting place – and this arises initially from the programme curriculum. The mentor will help channel ideas, enabling the student to identify specific areas of weakness, areas upon which to focus, where competence is to be developed. Each practicum will offer different learning opportunities and, as a mentor, my responsibility is making these known to the student and offering options in order that identified learning needs can be met. During the first weeks of the placement the learning plan is developed and this is a good way of working through options together. Since no two students are the same, it follows that no learning plan can be recycled.

Together the mentor and student will plan teaching and learning in line with curriculum outcomes and potential learning opportunities. The benefits of years of experience as a specialist practitioner come to the fore and there are many facets that will influence the quality of teaching:

- The complexities of patient assessment
- The influence of families and carers
- The pain endured in families who are 'going through it'
- The need and ability to stand in other people's shoes and to see through their eyes
- Knowing when to intervene and when intervention is inappropriate
- The importance of relationships based on trust
- The need for good communication skills
- Autonomy
- The influence of the nursing team upon the student
- Loyalty, respect, tolerance, trust, intuitive knowing – wisdom.

A clear teaching and learning plan is essential and joint learning contracts will provide further value. Further learning needs will be identifiable as the mentor evaluates student progress and teaching input throughout the practice placement.

The case load

An early task for the mentor is to set aside time in order to take the student through the student case-load and to be selective in planning visits where opportunities for learning exist. The case-load should (ideally) be neither too large and overwhelming nor so small that scope for learning is limited.

Gradually, and depending on their previous experiences, I enable the student to start to build up a case-load of patients and to take responsibility for the initial assessment and planning of care, with continued support and provision for feedback and critical analysis. Despite the student's apparent skills, it is vital that the mentor ensures that patient interventions are appropriate and fit for purpose and that the student is learning at the same time.

A fine line is drawn between promotion of student autonomy and the responsibility and accountability associated with case-load management. Specialist students, as registered nurses, are accountable for their actions but it is important to stress that as the case-load holder the mentor will be answerable in the event of harm or a formal complaint. This is one of the areas that can cause some degree of consternation as the mentor has to take a level of *knowledgeable* risk. By this I mean that at some stage we have to 'let go' otherwise the student will not develop relative autonomy of independent thought. The student can also learn from the risk-taking applied by the mentor. Having learned from experience, the specialist practitioner needs to know when rules can be broken – *taking* and not just managing risks (Wood 2000). Wisdom comes into play here, taking action based upon one's long experience of practice and student-awareness and knowing (almost intuitively) which course of action to take. This offers us an example of the 'swampy-lowlands' described by Schön (1991, p.42):

> '... or shall [the practitioner] descend to the swamp where he can engage the most important and challenging problems if he is willing to forsake technical rigor.'

If the case-load is inappropriate, too large or too small, it might be useful to talk to colleagues, to examine *their* case-loads and to make changes in order to expand or to reduce the content, thereby providing more scope for learning. Patients with more complex nursing needs or with a need for unpractised role-expansion may be 'shared' by the student and other, experienced practitioners. It is good for students to work alongside other practitioners and to experience different approaches.

Sometimes case-load pressures and other factors create difficulties and hinder teaching and learning. In the real world of practice we all need to prioritise and to make quick decisions about time and case-load management. Theoretically, student understanding of how staff cope under pressure is good experience, but students cannot thrive under stressed conditions for protracted periods. If there are on-going staffing problems then action has to be taken; it is all too easy to become reliant on a good student who is able to offer a solution by 'just getting on with it'. Students are in the placement to learn; it is the responsibility of the mentor to ensure that they are not exploited. If problems are not resolved, or in the case of health problems with the mentor, it may be necessary to take more drastic action and to consider moving the student to another area.

Professional, legal and ethical issues

Registered nurses are responsible for ensuring that they safeguard the inter-ests of their clients at all times. This responsibility encompasses delegation to other members of the health care team (UKCC 1999). It is important that patients and their families are aware of the status of the student and that they are able to make informed choices about the care they will receive. Equally important is the need to ask permission before assuming that individuals will receive students, however well qualified, into their home and into an existing nurse-patient relationship.

By and large patients *should* benefit from nurses' expansion of roles as this enables us to provide a more comprehensive and more patient-sensitive system of health care. It will be necessary to adhere to the policy of the employing authority; some are happy for expanded roles to be developed and used throughout the period of preparation for the specialist practitioner award, but not all are, so do check and adhere to your own Trust policies. UKCC guidelines must be followed (UKCC 1992a,b).

Student-mentor relationship

Schön (1987) talks of 'sharing our artistry' learning and reflecting together. The student might be inspired by the mentor but sometimes the reverse can happen. New ideas and innovative approaches to care serve to inspire the mentor and this is one of the 'mysteries' to be touched upon in the world of education. Dialogue between student, mentor and the university is important. If things are going well, it is good that all are aware; it is even more important to face any problems together – the timing is crucial. Any problems should be dealt with as soon as they arise; there is nothing to be gained by sweeping under the carpet issues which are beginning to create discomfort or interfering with student progress. A responsible and student-sensitive approach *must* be offered by the mentor.

Sometimes there will be difficulties. There may be a mismatch of teaching and learning styles between the student and mentor. This can be remedied provided the problem is picked up at an early stage; left unaddressed the student's learning will be impaired. It is important to set aside time to talk and to listen to one another. Often problems can be resolved by reviewing the learning contract and setting achievable goals within a short time-scale. Evaluation of progress will enable the mentor and student to discover ways in which future learning can be planned and achieved. If there are more unmanageable problems, a change of placement and mentor might be indi-cated; but this action needs to be taken at an early stage and any decision would involve staff from the HEI.

Reflective practice

Kate joined the team as a district nurse student. One of her first solo visits was to a single mother suffering from inoperable cancer. Some two or three weeks later I discovered that she was so upset by the situation that she had become over-involved with the family, her visits extending to her own time and even baby-sitting on one occasion. The children were well supported by their grandparents, but they themselves were unable to cope with their daughter's terminal condition.

In a reflective session, Kate started to talk about terminal illness and its impact upon the family; as she spoke she began to break down and I realised that she was completely out of her depth. There were a number of issues that she had not discussed with me because she had become so involved and felt unable to share her feelings and fears. I realised right away that I had not been supportive and that I should have spent time with Kate following her primary assessment visit. The workload had become overwhelming and there had been enormous pressure on our resources; I hadn't taken the time to discuss the visit with Kate. Three weeks had passed and Kate had seemed keen to visit this patient; she didn't highlight any problems and I had other issues to deal with, as well as staff sickness.

I suggested that we visited the patient together next day to jointly review Kate's assessment, taking into account any new problems. I would delegate some of my own visits in order to free-up some time. We had a long critical discussion about palliative care and I suggested that firstly, Kate should take a step back, in fairness to herself and the other patients in her care. I asked Kate about involving the wider community team and suggested that the community Macmillan nurse might be helpful. Kate seemed relieved. She had already suggested this but her suggestion hadn't gone down very well. The family had stated Kate herself would be 'their' nurse and she disclosed that this had, at the time, boosted her ego. I suggested that perhaps we could discuss this with the family next day. Kate realised that she had become out of her depth and felt foolish. I, in turn, came to realise that I had not acted in a responsible way in allowing the situation to develop. This turned out to be a clear illustration of critical review, in which new problems are discovered and appropriate action can be jointly planned and undertaken.

Case study 19.1 Reflection: a beneficial process for student and mentor

Time spent working alongside the mentor enables the student to ask, 'What have I learned from this experience?' or 'How would I change this action next time?'. The process of reflection motivates students when they look back at prior learning needs and their new-found skills and competence. This can be a real encouragement for students struggling to maintain vision and trying to remain focused on academic work and the development of practice and leadership skills. Reflection offers opportunities to continually re-evaluate, and to learn jointly.

Paul was finding difficulty in organising his time around patient care, record-keeping, clinics and staff-contact sessions. He arrived late and flustered at the GP surgery, having met an unexpected problem at his last patient visit. Also he told me he felt unable to complete his paperwork on time and this was adding to his anxiety. Earlier that week I had overheard a conversation between team members that Paul's studies were getting him down and that one of his tutors was overloading the students with work. I knew that Paul had some stresses at home which he had already discussed with me but this news had startled me. As far as I knew, Paul was unaware of my having overheard the conversation about his course concerns.

I reassured Paul and worked with him in the clinic. When the last patient had gone I spent time with him and explained that this is the 'real world' of district nursing and that all district nurses are faced with often agonising decision-making about organisation of work and documentation. Later that day, in a reflective session, Paul suggested that we looked at ways of improving his performance. Since the beginning of his placement he had demonstrated good potential but was aware that his organisation skills needed to be developed. Through a process of reflection he began to discover that he often took too much on-board and that he was unable to continue working in this way. Paul realised that his management skills were weak and that he lacked confidence in delegation. He felt embarrassed to ask others to take visits from him in order to complete his assessment documents and keep on top of other essential paperwork. I reassured him that, like other team members, he would gather new problems throughout the day, some of which would need immediate action. He asked me to help him develop the skills he would need; Paul realised that he needed to discuss his struggles with other team members. I asked Paul about his problems at home and he assured me that things were beginning to improve. After a pause he disclosed his doubts about his course and whether he had the staying-power to see it through. He shared some of his concerns about the volume of written work that was coming his way.

Paul needed support and encouragement. We chatted through his problems and I suggested he tried to prioritise them in order to deal with them in an objective way. He reassured me that his personal struggles weren't hindering his studies. I asked him if it would help to set up a meeting with his course leader and Paul thought this might be useful. Paul already knew that he could ask for an extension with his course work but didn't really want to fall further behind. He seemed to have a number of concerns and realised that he needed to get to the bottom of these himself. I too had concerns for him but realised that I was limited in my ability to deal with his problems.

Case study 19.2 Reflection: enabling student progress

If appropriate skills are not demonstrated, then the responsibility is on the mentor to act accordingly. Spending more time with the student is an obvious starting point, finding out if there is a problem that might be dealt with in some other way, going back to basics or finding an alternative strategy for teaching and learning. With the student's consent, the mentor might arrange to meet with university teachers. New goals might be set and perhaps a re-visiting of prior learning. Although most problems can be dealt with and solutions found (sometimes from the student), there will always be exceptions. A reflective approach is always helpful.

Supporting students throughout and beyond the academic year

Research undertaken with district nurses in the Tameside and Glossop area demonstrated the need for greater support in practice and education (Cavanagh 1998). Since 1997 I have been privileged to facilitate support and supervision sessions for specialist practitioner students. Meeting together on a monthly basis throughout the academic year has provided them with opportunities to discuss issues important to them, in a non-threatening environment. Reflective skills have been developed through these group sessions; better evaluation of their own performance within the system of education has been a positive outcome. Evaluation has been positive with the pilot cohort continuing into group supervision as newly qualified specialist practitioners and with different issues to debate as the transition is made from student to practitioner. One of the most interesting aspects has been the richness of the group environment brought about by the mix of disciplines (district nurse and health visitor students).

Summary

Juggling the role and responsibilities is the crux of the mentor role and I would challenge anyone to explain how this is done! So many roles within the one role, such a complex web, but perhaps this is what makes it all so worthwhile. I think that there are parallels between the caring role and the mentoring role, and mysteries that intertwine to create a tapestry most rich. Often problems have no clear solutions and there might be question marks even after the problem has been identified and addressed. Sometimes, problems that seem initially complex have a way of resolving themselves but this is not usually the case. One of the most meaningful lessons to be learned in mentoring is to expect the unexpected.

Opportunities for new approaches in practice will be offered as our vision for primary care is realised. Students may be less inhibited in their thinking and freer to consider new strategies than ourselves. So, if together we might somehow capture this enthusiasm and harness innovative thinking, there will be great potential for new practitioners to make a real impact upon primary care.

Chapter 20

Navigating Practice: Challenges and Opportunities

Joanne Bennett

Just before the end of the book, Joanne Bennett raises some 'wicked' issues for mentors (and all practitioners) to consider. In essence this is about refusing to stand still but rather moving forward as responsible, knowledgeable practitioners who are employed to provide quality health and health care. Moving toward better health and health care practices also ensures that the preparation students enjoy in practice will develop concurrently. But the needs of students cannot be presumed to occur simply by good practice in practice; mentors have the added responsibility of developing their teaching and facilitating role

---

Introduction

The complexity of professional practice and the challenges faced by those involved in the education of future community specialist practitioners have been central themes throughout this book. The challenge of educating future specialist practitioners is no easy task given that the problems encountered by professionals on an almost daily basis rarely have simple solutions that fall within the province of a single professional group, let alone one organisation. Specialist practitioners are frequently confronted with the diverse and complex problems and issues of the service user which cut across health, social care, housing, education and the environment (to name but a few). Any hope of finding a solution to many of these problems requires a very different way of working to that which is currently taking place. The intention of this chapter is to draw together some of the strands of this book through exploring the nature of the problems faced by practitioners, together with the implications of this on the preparation of future professionals. Although many of the issues are raised and discussed in a much broader context than mentorship, they clearly impact on the current and future delivery of practice and education.

Reflecting on the issues

There is a growing recognition by government that many of the needs of service users are becoming increasingly diverse. The Government is attempting to address this through a series of reforms which aim to put the service user and their specific needs at the centre of care delivery, which is based on partnership and integration of services. This is made explicit in the eighth principle of *The NHS Plan* (DoH 2000a) which states:

'The health and social care system must be shaped around the needs of the patient, not the other way round. The NHS will develop partnerships and co-operation at all levels of care – between patients, their carers and families and NHS staff; between the health and social care sector; between different government departments; between the public sector, voluntary organisations and private providers in the provision of NHS services – to ensure a patient centred service.'

The plan also suggests that the NHS has a patchy record in demonstrating its ability to look beyond health care to health, arguing that:

'The wider inability to forge effective partnerships with local government, business and community organisations has inhibited the NHS' ability to prevent ill health and tackle health inequalities . . . This fault line needs to be addressed.'

(DoH 2000a, p. 29)

The Government's approach to addressing these deficits has been 'top-down', one of high control and low trust, with partnership behaviour being specified (Henwood & Hudson, 2000). These authors go on to suggest that this approach needs to be balanced by a bottom-up perspective which focuses on front-line staff who are left to put the Government agenda into practice, arguing that if we are to find any resolution to complex problems, or what are often referred to as 'wicked issues', new partnerships must be forged. Simi-larly, the world of education needs to reflect the changes that are taking place (or are about to take place) in practice and in doing so ensure that future practitioners are prepared for their role.

What are 'wicked issues'?

According to Clarke and Stewart (2000), the term 'wicked issues' is used to describe a policy problem without an obvious or established solution; a problem which does not sit conveniently within the remit or responsibility of any one organisation. They describe how the phrase was first used by Horst Rittel and Melvin Webber who said:

'We are calling them "wicked" not because these properties are themselves ethically deplorable. We use the term "wicked" in a meaning akin to that "malignant" (in contrast to "benign") or "vicious" (like a circle) or "tricky" (like a leprechaun) or "aggressive" (like a lion, in contrast to the docility of a lamb) (Rittel and Webber, 1973, p.160).'

In other words, 'wicked issues' are those where:

- 'the problem itself is hard to define;
- causal chains are difficult (if not impossible) to unravel;
- complex inter-dependencies are involved'.

(Henwood & Hudson 2000, p. 47)

It is becoming clear that many of the problems faced by practitioners from a variety of professional backgrounds could easily fall into this category of 'wicked issues', particularly given the increasing emphasis being placed on the role of front-line workers in policy implementation. Lipsky (1980) proposed that public policy is best understood through the daily encounters of 'street-level bureaucrats' (e.g. doctors, nurses, social workers), not on the top-level floor suites of high ranking administrators. The central thrust of his argument was that street-level bureaucrats have enormous power, which they can use to control service users as well as maintain their own autonomy. However, he discusses this in the context of the difficult position they find themselves in, rather than in terms of power abuse. Due to working conditions, they encounter situations on a daily basis where demand for services far exceeds supply. They are consequently forced to devise strategies to cope, which in turn result in the making of public policy. The importance he places upon professionals is highlighted in the following statement:

'Citizens directly experience government through them, and their actions *are* the policies provided by government in important respects'.

(Lipsky 1980, p. xvi)

Tackling the 'wicked issues'

What this points to is an urgent need for practitioners, service managers (from a variety of organisations, professional and non-professional backgrounds), the public and education to work together to resolve the 'wicked' issues which are part of everyday life in practice and education. The top-down approach to policy implementation needs to be balanced by a bottom-up perspective which focuses on local problems and local solutions (Henwood & Hudson 2000). Any hopes of finding these solutions will be dependent on very different ways of thinking and working that cut across internal and external boundaries. Clarke and Stewart (2000) suggest that resolution is likely to occur when we start to go through the iterative process of learning, trying and learning. Similarly, the use of a reflective framework, such as that described in Chapter 5, may provide a useful approach for this. Regardless of the process adopted there is a requirement to work through people, the front-line workers, who are responsible for policy in action.

The different ways of thinking and working that are required to move towards some sort of resolution pose major challenges for existing patterns of service organisation and management, existing models of service delivery and existing educational provision. The remainder of this chapter will explore some of these challenges prior to examining *some* of the strategies that may be of use to service managers, practitioners, practice educators, mentors and academics at the cutting edge of change.

The context

The constraints imposed on all of those involved in the development and implementation of specialist practitioner courses are numerous. Mary Dunning provided insight into this in Chapter 3 where she highlights the complexity of developing and maintaining standards in a curriculum. Among the multitude of factors to be taken into consideration when developing a curriculum are:

- The requirements of the UKCC and ENB which relate to the standard, kind and content of courses (see Chapter 1)
- Internal and external quality standards that must be met
- The requirements of local stakeholders
- The involvement and views of service users
- The involvement and views of practitioners and managers
- The provision of suitable placement areas
- The support of the local workforce development confederation
- National policy and its influence on curriculum content (see Chapter 2)
- The skill mix of academic staff needed to deliver the curriculum
- The preparation of teachers (practice and academic)
- Workforce planning issues
- Cost effectiveness of the course
- An innovative and up-to-date curriculum
- The total length of the course.

Every effort has been made by those involved in the development and implementation of specialist practitioner courses to prepare practitioners who are responsive, adaptable and multi-skilled and who are equipped with skills in life-long learning. This is evident in many of the chapters of this book where authors describe the innovative strategies and approaches that they have used in an attempt to encourage practitioners to be critical thinkers and to work in very different ways from in the past. Although there have been considerable moves forward in the preparation of these specialists for their role (see Chapter 1) many of the constraints to further developing aspects of specialist practice, including partnership working and inter-professional education, remain and a radical rethink is needed. However, before moving on to explore this in more detail consideration will be given to some of the challenges which must be addressed to improve the quality of service delivery in practice and education. Although some of these are outside of the remit of both the mentor and practice educator, they clearly influence and impact on each of these roles, the learning environment and the student's learning experience.

Challenges

Organisational structures and boundaries

Any movement towards a resolution of the complex or 'wicked' issues involves working across organisational boundaries and drawing many organisations into the frame. However, as Clarke and Stewart (2000) point out, organisations cannot work effectively together if they do not work effectively within themselves. *The NHS Plan* appears to assume that demarcations and boundaries between professions can be overcome by putting a range of professionals within a Care Trust. Henwood and Hudson (2000) rightly indicate that this is a simplistic view, which becomes evident if inter-professional working within the NHS in general and within primary health care teams in particular is examined, citing evidence which highlights professional schisms in three areas of the NHS: nursing-nursing (Armstrong *et al.* 1994; Wood *et al.* 1994; MacDonald *et al.* 1997); nursing-medicine (Conway *et al.* 1995; Robinson *et al.* 1993; Wiles *et al.* 1994); and medicine-medicine (Jenkins-Clarke *et al.* 1997). Henwood and Hudson (2000) conclude by arguing that inter-professional working has been more of an aspiration than a reality, as this would involve:

- 'sharing knowledge;
- respect for the autonomy of different professional groups;
- surrender of professional territory where necessary;
- a shared set of values concerning appropriate responses to shared definitions of need'.

(p.16)

Furthermore, values, attitudes and bias are socially and institutionally embedded (Dalley 1993). The Government's agenda has been projected onto a history of differences in professional cultures and ideologies, resulting in strained relationships between staff within and external to organisations, which has not been helped through policy that encouraged competition at the expense of collaboration.

Nevertheless, the education and continuing professional development of professionals is central to the socialisation process. Although this is widely recognised within higher education institutes, only a few have made any real moves towards addressing this. For example, Kingston University and St George's Hospital Medical School in the UK provide a common foundation programme for radiographers, physiotherapists, scientists, nurses and doctors (DoH 2000e, p.27). Whilst it is acknowledged that there are valuable lessons to be learned from such experiences, two important issues must be noted. First, academic staff have been through the same socialisation process themselves; and second, the university setting plays only a small part in the socialisation process – clinical placements and work experience on qualifying are of major significance.

The academic structure within some universities does little to break down internal professional barriers. The location of discipline specialists within schools, the need to align funding streams to that school's activity and the moves to increase student numbers while at the same time reduce the number of academic staff, are all doing little to break down professional barriers and promote or encourage different ways of thinking and working. Questions must be asked of a system which has set a demanding agenda for professionals and all of those involved in their education and development, but at the same time is expecting more student numbers with fewer academic staff. Multi-professional learning is not about 100 students in a lecture theatre being 'talked at' by the teacher, it is about learning together and from each other and perhaps more importantly developing respect and trust. The possibility of this with such large class sizes is questionable.

The structures and boundaries that currently exist within NHS Trusts and General Practice also serve to reinforce professional identities and boundaries and often inhibit partnership working and multi-professional education (Henwood & Hudson 2000; DoH 2000a). It has already been pointed out that this is both internal and external to organisations. The strained relationship that often exists between the NHS and social care providers is arguably exacerbated by health care being free at the point of delivery, yet access to some elements of social care being financially variable. Furthermore, community specialist practice in many areas is characterised by heavy case-loads, limited skill mix in some disciplines (e.g. health visiting and general practice nursing), major organisational change with the development of PCGs and PCTs, and the need for continuing professional development to meet the changing requirements of the role (e.g. evidence-based practice, national service frameworks, quality and audit), which all leaves little time to develop and promote new ways of working. The publication of the standards for the preparation of mentors and teachers of nursing, midwifery and health visiting (UKCC 2000a) will arguably add to these demands as they have major implications for the professional development of many existing mentors. If we are serious about moving this agenda forward, practitioners require protected time and investment to facilitate advances in practice, to develop new roles, to work across organisational boundaries and develop partnership-working, and to facilitate the education and development of themselves and others.

Skill mix

It is essential that a robust review of existing skill mix in both practice and education is undertaken in order to determine the education and development needs of existing staff as well as the needs of future specialist practitioners. The importance of adopting an integrated and inter-professional approach to this is crucial if we are serious about meeting service user needs. This is recognised in *A Health Service of all talents: Developing the NHS Workforce* (DoH 2000c, 2.1) which states: 'In the case of healthcare its fundamental purpose is to ensure that there are sufficient staff available with the right skills to deliver high quality care to patients'.

Many existing community specialist practitioners qualified when courses were at certificate or diploma level. They therefore hold the title of a specialist practitioner, not the award (see Chapter 1). The many years of clinical expertise that this group has developed is invaluable to the profession. Despite this, many of these groups have had little opportunity to develop the knowledge base commensurate with the 'new' role. Recent work with the entire group of district nursing specialist practitioners in a local NHS community trust highlighted the extent of this. Among the professional development needs identified were knowledge and skills in health need assessment, research appreciation, managing change, policy analysis, quality and audit and chairing meetings. These findings were reinforced through an education and training needs analysis that a colleague and myself conducted with general practice nurses in a local PCG.

Realistic and local strategies must be found to address workforce planning, and the continuing professional development of staff, which must be based on the needs of the service. Of equal importance is the provision of protected time for study, which does not rely on the continual 'goodwill' of practitioners. Alongside this is the need to review the skill mix of academic staff. A review of any nursing department within a UK university will demonstrate limited numbers of academic staff with expertise and qualifications in primary health care. This seems a paradox given the policy focus in this area and the current emphasis given to primary care in both pre-registration and post-registration curricula.

Funding streams

A further barrier to inter-disciplinary education is the separate funding streams that exist for professional groups. This has served to inhibit inter-disciplinary education and creative solutions to the needs of service users. In an attempt to address this it has been suggested that an integrated approach to levy funding needs to be adopted, which facilitates rather than inhibits inter-disciplinary education. The proposal is that the workforce confederation will explore this as part of workforce planning (DoH 2000c).

Policy agenda

Policy implementation is an integral part of the role of service managers, practitioners and educationalists. Given the demands placed on the specialist practitioner role, and the embryonic nature of information technology facilities in some areas of primary care, it is often difficult for these practitioners to keep abreast of policy change and legislation influencing and directing care delivery. In addition to this, the translation of national and local policy into practice is a skill that many specialists have not had the opportunity or time to acquire. The development of national guidelines and centres to assist with some elements of this are no doubt helpful, but are dependent on access to, and skills in, information technology. Unless this is addressed there is a risk that the policy implementation gap will continue. This problem is also mirrored within some higher education institutes, which lack a clear strategy for policy analysis in terms of the implications for practice and education.

Involving the public

Local solutions need to be found to local problems (Henwood & Hudson 2000). In order to do this it is essential that we involve the public in a meaningful way. This is central to our understanding of the real problems faced by service users and to the development of a variety of approaches to meeting need. Some areas of nursing have demonstrated more success with involving the public than others (e.g. mental health nursing). Sharing of success stories from other health and social care providers may be a useful starting point for those who have to date done no more than pay lip service to public involvement in this area.

Towards a new approach

The problems highlighted above are probably familiar to many managers, practitioners, mentors and educationalists. It is clear from this that there is a need for:

- The recognition that understanding is at its best partial and that uncertainty is acceptable
- Holistic thinking, encompassing the interactions of a wide variety of activities, behaviours and attitudes
- The capacity to accept different approaches, perspectives and styles to working, to refuse to be trapped by the obvious and conventional
- Being inclusive, the ability to involve a wide range of organisations and agencies as well as the public in developing solutions and responses
- The ability to think and work in completely new ways which involve interacting, accepting different perspectives and approaches, risk-taking, reflecting, evaluating and learning from experiences
- The ability to learn from actions.

(Adapted from Clarke & Stewart 2000)

The enormity of such change cannot be over-emphasised and a planned and staged programme must be developed. It would be impossible here to explore the implications of this in detail, so this chapter will focus on some possible actions that could be taken by front-line workers who are at the forefront of service delivery and practice development; mentors and practice educators fall within this group.

Change at a local level must be targeted and realistic in its time-scale and cost. What follows are suggestions for debate which have emerged from discussions with colleagues, analysis of policy and reflecting on my current activities with community trusts, PCGs, PCTs and to a lesser extent the local council. Like most of us, my understanding is partial and this may be evident to some readers with different ideas and areas of expertise to myself. However, unless we begin to articulate our ideas, share and engage in debate with others and further develop strategies for drawing on the collective expertise of professionals and non-professionals, we may be at risk of providing more of the same in both education and practice.

Development of a task force

Existing organisational design is premised on the need to focus, simplify and order, to operate efficiently, effectively and economically. While such an approach is deemed to be of value in dealing with easily identified problems with simple solutions that fall into the remit of one organisation, deficits become apparent when attempts are made to deal with the more complex issues and problems that cut across organisational boundaries. Within such systems day-to-day work and routine activities have a tendency to overcrowd the more complex and non-routine, which can easily be forgotten or given periodic attention when time and workload permit (Clarke & Stewart 2000). Within this type of system we are at risk from perpetuating linear thinking by failing to look beyond the obvious. For example, health promotion is an area that involves the NHS, local government and other organisations, yet this is rarely demonstrated through the collective involvement of representatives from these organisations in the planning and delivery of activity in this area in either practice or education.

Through consideration of the above, one approach worthy of debate is the development of a local task force, which involves a range of organisations and the public to seek solutions to the 'wicked issues'. Success of such an approach is dependent on many factors, including protected time, adequate funding, commitment to the issues, and the ability and willingness to share expertise, knowledge and experiences, accept different perspectives, learn from each other and take risks. Of equal importance is the identification of a visionary leader who is committed to the development of different ways of thinking and working. Although it is essential that such a group has adequate clout, this does not imply that the leader should be the most senior person; leadership qualities do not necessarily equate with those of a manager.

Although many of us may welcome the opportunity to be involved in developing new approaches to service delivery, the reality is that day-to-day maintenance activity must continue. Adopting this type of approach would enable the majority to continue with this whilst at the same time allowing those with dedicated time opportunities to explore the 'wicked issues', share ideas and develop and test new models of service delivery based on service user needs. If successful, this could then be fed back into the system and become part of the mainstream activity. Among the many issues that would need to be considered is that of communication across and within organisations to prevent staff feeling marginalised. The raising of awareness of 'wicked issues' also implies a commitment to education and training, which would emerge from the needs of practice.

Focus

The focus on 'wicked issues' is growing, and we need to begin to understand the nature of those that are evident locally. Given the finite nature of resources, some priorities and parameters must be set to prevent us 'drowning'. A starting point for this could be an analysis of the health and social needs of the local community. While there will already be a considerable amount of relevant information available within organisations, attempts must be made to integrate this information. With this in mind, boundaries need to be agreed and mechanisms established to collate, analyse and rectify any gaps in this data. Only then can local priority areas be determined based on local need. The relationship of this to HImP priorities and national targets must also be explored.

While this information may be helpful in determining areas of greatest need, its value in enhancing understanding of 'wicked issues' is debatable as it does not necessarily help to uncover the real problems and experiences of service users, professionals and non-professionals. One technique, which may prove to be of value, is critical incident analysis (see Chapter 5). Greater understanding will hopefully be achieved through the process of gathering the experiences (positive and negative) of service users, professionals and non-professionals and analysing them through the use of a reflective framework. Only when understanding has been enhanced can new ways of working be developed, tested and evaluated. Although I have not had experience of using this technique in the way I am suggesting here, a colleague and myself have successfully used it with a group of GPs' community nurse managers, specialist practitioners and non-professional health authority staff, as a strategy to develop and improve practice. Alternatively, an action research framework such as that described by Hart and Bond (1995) may prove useful, as the focus for the development is practice and it is action dominated and based on a partnership approach. Through either process, the educational and development needs of practitioners will emerge from practice rather than education.

Continuing professional development needs

Greater understanding of the 'wicked issues' has implications for the way in which we meet the continuing professional development needs of staff. The Chief Medical Officer's Report (Calman 1998) on the future of continuing professional development (CPD) in primary care offers a useful framework to plan development needs. Here it is envisaged that practice-based education plans are derived from the needs of *all* practice staff which, in turn, are matched to the objectives of the practice as well as local and national objectives (which is what is suggested above). In other words, personal learning and development must be linked to the needs of the organisation. Furthermore, education and development must be broader than the acquisition of clinical and technical skills, encompassing the concept of life-long learning. This should be built into all the levels of PCG functioning and should take place across professional and organisational boundaries. With this in mind, future education and development must be flexible, targeted and relevant to the needs of service users and the organisation, accredited (if required) and inter-professional.

Many attempts are already under way to develop different approaches to meeting the continuing professional development needs of existing professionals and non-professionals in primary care. For example, the University of Northumbria has appointed a principal lecturer in primary care to work with partner organisations to explore different ways of meeting identified need. A number of projects have emerged from this appointment, all of which take place in the workplace. A central tenet of all of the activity is the development of a culture of learning where expertise is shared; problem-based and solution-focused approaches to practice development which avoid blame are adopted; teamwork and enhanced understanding of each other's role and contribution are promoted; and enhancement in the quality of the service delivered is sought. The popularity of this approach is evident through the growing number of requests from community trusts and PCGs. Furthermore, the accreditation of work-based learning is viewed by many community nurse managers as one of the possible strategies to assist existing specialist practitioners, mentors and practice educators to acquire the knowledge and skills to meet their changing role (see Chapter 1 for new standards).

The specialist practitioner curriculum

The overall impact of the suggested changes on the preparation of future specialist practitioners can only be positive. The development of new partnerships, educational strategies delivered in practice and the promotion of a learning organisation will hopefully enhance the learning environment and student experience through enabling the students to cross organisational boundaries and develop new approaches to service delivery in ways that have not been possible in the past. This will also be dependent on the skills and attributes of the practice educator who has a central role to play in the co-ordination and facilitation of the students' experience. However, developments are varying in terms of scale and pace between and within organisations and as yet there has been limited involvement from wider organisations in the process. It will therefore take some time before some of these practices become part of mainstream activity. There are many reasons for this which include the need to develop inter-professional learning and working within the NHS, the need to overcome the difficulties imposed through separate funding streams and the logistics of getting staff together at the same time, whilst maintaining service delivery. Although the developments are in their infancy, and longer-term evaluation needs to take place on their effectiveness, initial response from managers and participants has been positive. The university is currently exploring ways in which to address issues of skill mix and is increasing the capacity of academic staff in primary care to further promote the development and delivery of practice-led work-based initiatives.

New developments and opportunities in practice must be reflected in theoretical and practical components of the specialist practitioner curriculum, which ideally should develop in tandem to avoid perpetuating the theory-practice gap (examples of this have already been highlighted in Chapter 2 where I described the dilemmas in moving towards a population approach to public health). Although, there is no doubt that innovative approaches to the development of practitioners who are equipped with skills in critical thinking, problem-solving and life-long learning are integral to many existing courses, this being reflected in the strategies and approaches to learning and assessment described in this book, the development of a specialist practitioner curriculum which *truly* addresses the inter-professional nature of practice remains at the discussion stage for many.

The main areas of shared learning are confined to the core elements of specialist practitioner courses, where delivery is usually with other professionals undertaking study in a different area of specialist practice. The way in which we begin to address the challenge of, for example, how to promote problem-based approaches to learning, which are inter-disciplinary, in class sizes of between 80–100 remains to be seen. The logistics of doing this requires a radical review of skill mix, current course structure and indeed the requirements of different regulating bodies (among others). Solutions to this are complex and will not happen overnight. Nevertheless, front-line staff must continue to develop ideas and strategies in an attempt to take this agenda forward.

Given the continual emphasis placed on the importance of education being derived from the needs of practice, consideration could perhaps be given to increasing the emphasis of work-based learning in the curriculum. This would help to ensure that the learning was targeted and relevant to the needs of practice. The success of this type of initiative would again be dependent on the knowledge and skills of the mentor or practice educator and their ability to forge links and work in partnership with others. Furthermore, while strategies such as critical incident analysis and problem-based learning are becoming less tenable within the classroom environment with large groups of students, they can be encouraged in practice, with smaller groups of students and indeed qualified staff. This would create further opportunities for mentors, practice educators and academic staff to work in partnership to facilitate learning based on the realities of practice.

Conclusion

The context in which practice teaching is taking place is extremely complex. The demands placed on the specialist practitioner from government, management, the profession, education and the public (as well as others) can at times be overwhelming. Indeed, review of current and future expectations of those undertaking this role suggests that demands will increase, particularly given the importance of 'street level' staff in policy implementation, local and national, internal and external to the organisation. Success will clearly be dependent on the knowledge, skills and attitudes of this group. This implies the need for increased recognition of the importance of the role of specialist practitioners, mentors and practice educators in meeting the changing requirements of the service user, together with real investment in their continuing professional development, an essential pre-requisite to fulfilling the role. Of equal importance is the need for investment in strategies that aim to improve relationships between front-line staff and encourage different key players to think and work in different ways.

Chapter 21
Concluding Comments

Judith Canham and Joanne Bennett

In this book, contributors' reflections on the mentor role range from challenging to difficult and hard, though interestingly none feel it is impossible or an unwelcome addition to the practitioner role. The art of the role appears to include collaborating, combining, prioritising and adapting whilst at the same time being resourceful, multi-skilled, patient and committed! Although 'dedicated' is out of favour (when applied to nursing) there can be no doubt that in order to undertake the role of mentor dedication to the concept of specialist practice education and furtherance of specialisms is required. However, dedication in the form of protected time to undertake the role is usually missing and most mentors will continue to find that mentoring is additional to their practitioner role.

It is clear that considering the dual role of the mentor and the need to develop the specialist student's professional practice within a limited time-scale, the sheer weight of theory and policy may be considered daunting. The advantage for mentors is that as they are immersed in practice, those policies, theories and standards that directly influence community (and all) health practices can be immediately recognised for their relevance to a specific professional world.

At present there is little evidence to demonstrate the benefits of specialist community practice education and this must be a cause for concern to teachers in HEI and mentors in practice. Nursing and health visiting have been subject to much postulation regarding their ability, through education, to provide health care and health empowerment to the UK population. As there is little evidence to support the benefits of specialist practice to health and health care, preparation for these roles may be questioned.

It is more than possible that through the appropriate use of relevant learning, teaching and assessment strategies, mentors will be able to facilitate the professional progress of specialist practitioners able to accept responsibility for their own continuing professional development, promote change, reflect and receive and contribute to clinical supervision. If these attributes are seen, through research focused on neophyte specialist practitioners, to have effect on both practice and service users, education in both HEI and practice will have fulfilled its obligation.

It is interesting that though the concept of HEI-mentor collaboration is propounded, contributors rarely articulate how it is facilitated. As mentors are facilitating up to 50% of an educational programme, it is imperative that they are closely involved with ensuring the quality of *their* programme. It is true that HEIs are subject to exceedingly pedantic and inflexible quality direction (some self-imposed), but as the intention is to provide a high quality educational experience, from application to the award ceremony (and sometimes beyond), perhaps the detail of the quality process can be excused. The expertise of mentors and their articulation of practice can enable the weighty and complex HEI quality process to:

(1) Be more centred on real-life practice through contributions to programme committees and quality review
(2) Support the primacy of practice and encourage practice classification
(3) Confirm that, and how, taught principles are transferred to practice, and vice versa.

Preparing this book has been as challenging as the mentor role – prioritising, agreeing an appropriate degree of standardisation and trying to be all things to all people. We know that some issues have not been included but what we really hope is that this book will enable your development and go some small way to helping the mentor survive and prosper.

References

Abraham, M. (1990) Promoting Children's Health. *Nursing Standard*, **4** (21) 6–7.

Alavi, C. & Cattoni, J. (1995) Good nurse, bad nurses ... *Journal of Advanced Nursing*, **21**, 344–9.

Andrews, S. (1991) *Facing the Challenge in Community Nurse Education*. Queen's Nursing Institute, London.

Appleton, J. (1999) Assessing vulnerability in families In: *Research issues in community nursing* (ed. J. McIntosh). MacMillan, Basingstoke.

Appleton, J. & Cowley, S. (eds) (2000) *The Search for Health Needs: Research for Health Visiting Practice*. MacMillan, Basingstoke.

Arber, S. & Ginn, J. (1995) 'Only connect': gender relations and aging. In: *Connecting Gender and Aging: A sociological approach* (eds S. Arber and J. Ginn). Open University Press, Buckingham.

Arendt, H. (1958) *The Human Condition*. University of Chicago Press, Chicago.

Arendt, H. (1977) *Between Past and Future*. Penguin Books, New York.

Armstrong, D., Taverbie, A. & Johnston, S. (1994) Job satisfaction among practice nurses in a health district. *Health and Social Care in the Community*, **2**, 279–82.

Atkins, S. & Murphy, K. (1993) Reflection: a review of the literature. *Journal of Advanced Nursing*, **18**, 1188.

Audit Commission (1999) *First Assessment: a review of district nursing services in England and Wales*. Audit Commission, London.

Ausubel, D. P. (1968) *Educational Psychology: a cognitive view*. Holt, Rinehart and Winston, New York.

Baillie, L. (1993) Factors affecting student nurses' learning in community placements: a phenomenological study. *Journal of Advanced Nursing*, **18**, 1043–53.

Bamford, M. & Warner, J. (1998) *Occupational Health Nurses Education and Training Needs to meet the New Public Health Agenda and Occupational Health Services contribution to meeting workforce planning requirements*. Unpublished Report commissioned by NHSE West Midlands.

Barker, P. (1998) Psychiatric nursing. In: *Clinical Supervision and Mentorship in Nursing*, 2nd edn, (Eds T. Butterworth, J.Faugier & P. Burnard). Thornes, Cheltenham.

Barry, D. (1999) Making reflection a rewarding and productive experience. *Nursing Times Learning Curve*, **3** (5) 2–3.

Beck, D.L.R. & Scrivastava, R. (1991) Perceived levels and sources of stress in baccalaureate students. *Journal of Nursing Education*, **30**, 127–33.

Benner, P. (1984) *From Novice to Expert: excellence and power in clinical nursing practice*. Addison-Wesley, California.

Bishop, V. (1998) Clinical supervision: what is it? In: *Clinical Supervision in Practice: some questions, answers and guidelines*, (ed. V. Bishop). MacMillan Press, London.

Bishop, V. (2000) Editorial. *Nursing Times Research*, **5** (3) 164.

Blomfield, R. & Hardy, S. (2000) Evidence-based nursing practice. In: *Evidence-Based Practice: A Critical Appraisal*, (eds L. Trinder & S. Reynolds). Blackwell Science, London.

Bond, M. & Holland, S. (1998) *Skills of Clinical Supervision for Nurses*. Open University Press, Buckingham.

Booth, K. & Luker, K. (1999) *A Practical Handbook for Community Health Nurses Working with Children and their Parents*. Blackwell Science, Oxford.

Botting, B. (ed.) (1995) *The Health of Our Children: decennial supplement*. HMSO, London.

Boud, D., Keogh, R. & Walker, D. (1985) Promoting reflection in learning. In: *Turning Experience into Learning* (eds D. Boud, R. Keogh & D. Walker). Kogan Page, London.

Bowers, L. (1996) Community psychiatric nurse education in the United Kingdom: 8 years of surveys and the issues raised. *Journal of Advanced Nursing*, **23**, 919–24.

Bowers, L. (1997) Mental health. In: *Community Care: Initial training and beyond* (ed. D. Skidmore). Arnold, London.

Boyd, E.M. & Fales, A.W. (1983) Reflective Learning; key to learning from experience. *Journal of Humanistic Psychology*, **23** (2) 99–117.

Brookfield, S. (1987) *Developing Critical Thinkers*. Open University Press, Buckingham.

Burnard, P. (1990) Critical Awareness in Nurse Education. *Nursing Standard* **4** (30) 32–4.

Butterworth, T. (1998) Clinical supervision as an emerging idea. In: *Clinical Supervision and Mentorship in Nursing*, 2nd edn, (eds T. Butterworth, J. Faugier & P. Burnard). Thornes, Cheltenham.

Butterworth, T. & Woods, D. I. (1998) *Clinical Governance and Clinical Supervision: working together to ensure safe and accountable practice*. The School of Nursing, Midwifery and Health Visiting, University of Manchester.

Calman, K.A. (1998) *Review of continuing professional development in General Practice*. Chief Medical Officer report. DoH, London.

Canham, J. (1991) *Policies, politics and change: the effects on continuing education. A study of Community Practice Teachers in the North Western Regional Health Authority*. MSc thesis, Manchester Metropolitan University.

Canham, J. (1998) Educational clinical supervision: meeting the needs of specialist community practitioner students and professional practice. *Nurse Education Today*, **18**, 394–8.

Carper, B. (1978) Fundamental patterns of knowing in nursing. *Advances in Nursing Science*, **1** (1) 13–23.

Castledine, G. (1994) Clinical supervision: a real aspiration? *British Journal of Nursing* **3** (16) 805.

Cavanagh, M. (1998) *District nurses' perceptions of continuing professional education*. BSc thesis, the Department of Health Care Studies, the Manchester Metropolitan University.

Cernick, K. & Evans, J. (1992) Developing competency objectives as a basis for planning and assessing health visiting practice in training. *Nurse Education Today*, **12**, 37–43.

Chalmers, H. (1999) *Guidance for peer review and observation process*. Marcet Series 11: Guides for staff: Paper 12. University of Northumbria.

Chambers, M.A. (1998) Some issues in the assessment of clinical practice: a review of the literature. *Journal of Clinical Nursing*, **7**, 201–208.

Clarke, M.L. (2000) Out of the wilderness and into the fold: the school nurse and child protection. *The Child Abuse Review*, **9**, 364–74.

Clarke, M. & Stewart, J. (2000) Handling the wicked issues. In: *Changing Practice in Health and Social Care* (eds C. Davies, L. Finlay & A. Bullman). Sage Publications, London.

Clifton, M., Brown, J. & Shaw, I. (1993) *Learning Disabilities and the Specialist Nurse.* SPSW Publishing. York.

Conway, M., Armstong, D. & Bickler, G. (1995) A corporate needs assessment fot the purchase of district nursing. *Public Health,* **109**, 337–45.

Cowley, S. (1995) In health visiting, a routine visit is one that has passed. *Journal of Advanced Nursing,* **22**, 276–84.

Cowley, S., Buttigieg, M. & Houston, A. (2000) *A First Steps Project to Scope the Current and Future Regulatory Issues for Health Visiting.* Unpublished report prepared for the United Kingdom Central Council for Nursing, Midwifery and Health Visiting. UKCC, London.

CPHVA (1998) *Healthy Futures: The Diversity of School Nursing.* Community Practitioners and Health Visitors Association, London.

CPHVA (1999) *National Framework for School Nursing Practice.* Community Practitioners and Health Visitors Association, London.

CPHVA (2000a) *School Nursing: a national framework for practice.* Community Practitioners and Health Visitors Association, London.

CPHVA (2000b) *Practice Educators Preparing for New Roles in the NHS.* Community Practitioner and Health Visitors Association, London

Craig, P.M. & Lyndsay, G.M. (2000) *Nursing for Public Health: population based health care.* Churchill Livingstone, London.

Crossley, N. (1996) *Intersubjectivity: the fabric of social becoming.* Sage, London.

Culley, L. & Genders, N. (1999) Parenting by people with learning disabilities: the educational needs of the community nurse. *Nurse Education Today,* **19**, 502–508.

Cust, J. (1996) A relational view of learning. *Nurse Education Today,* **16**, 256–66.

Dale, P., Douglas, M., Morrison, T. & Waters, J. (1986) *Dangerous Families. Assessment and treatment of child abuse.* Routledge, London.

Dalley, G. (1993) Professional ideology or organisational tribalism. In: *Health, Welfare and Practice: Reflecting on Roles and Relationships,* (eds. J. Walmsley, J. Reynolds, P. Shakespeare & R. Woolfe) Open University Press, Sage Publications, London.

Damant, M., Martin, C. & Openshaw. M.C. (1994) *Practice Nursing: stability and change.* Mosby, London.

Davies, S., Shepherd, B., Thompson, A. & Whittaker, K. (1995) *An Investigation into the Changing Educational Needs of Community Nurse, Midwives and Health Visitors in Relation to the Teaching, Supervising and Assessing of Pre- and Post-Registration Students.* English National Board, London.

Davis, B.D. (1990) How nurses learn and how to improve the learning environment. *Nurse Education Today,* **10**, 405–409.

Deacon, M. (1998) *The organisation of a mental health team.* M.Phil thesis. The University of Manchester.

DeBell, D. & Jackson, P. (2000) *School Nursing within the Public Health Agenda. A Strategy for Practice.* McMillan-Scott on behalf of Queens Institute of Nurses. London.

DfEE (1997) *The National Committee of Enquiry into Higher Education.* Department for Education and Employment, London.

DHSS (1977) The Report of the Committee on Nursing (the Briggs Report). HMSO, London.

DiCenso, A., Cullum, N. & Ciliska, D. (1998) Implementing evidence-based nursing: some misconceptions (editorial). *Evidence-Based Nursing,* **1**, 38–40.

Dimond, B. (1990) *Legal Aspects of Nursing*. Prentice Hall, London.

DoH (1989a) *Working for Patients*. Cmnd 555. HMSO, London.

DoH (1989b) *Caring for People*. Cmnd 849. HMSO, London.

DoH (1993) *Vision for the Future: the nursing, midwifery and health visiting contribution to health and health care*. NHSE, London.

DoH (1997a) *The New NHS: modern, dependable*. The Stationery Office, London.

DoH (1997b) *Report on the Review of the Nurses, Midwives and Health Visitors Act*. The Stationery Office, London.

DoH (1998a) *A First Class Service: Quality in the New NHS*. Department of Health, Leeds.

DoH (1998b) *Non-medical education and training (NMET) funding devolution to education consortia*. Health Service Circular (1998/044). Department of Health, London.

DoH (1998c) *Developing Primary Care Groups*. HSC 139, Department of Health, London.

DoH (1998d) *Health Improvement Programme: Planning for Better Health and Better Health Care*. HSC 167, Department of Health, London.

DoH (1998e) *The New NHS Modern and Dependable: Primary Care Groups: Delivering the Agenda*. HSC 228, Department of Health, London.

DoH (1998f) *Commissioning in the New NHS: Commissioning Services 1999–2000*. HSC 198, Department of Health, London.

DoH (1998g) *Partnership in Action: A discussion document*. The Stationery Office, London.

DoH (1999a) *Making a Difference*. The Stationery Office, London.

DoH (1999b) *Saving Lives: Our Healthier Nation*. The Stationery Office, London.

DoH (2000a) *The NHS Plan*. The Stationery Office, London.

DoH (2000b) *NHS R&D Funding Consultation Paper: NHS priorities and needs R&D funding*. The Stationery Office, London.

DoH (2000c) *A Health Service of all talents: developing the NHS workforce*. The Stationery Office, London.

DoH (2000d) (A. Cox & A. Bentovim) *The family assessment pack of questionnaires and scales*. The Stationery Office, London.

DoH (2000e) *Meeting the Challenge: A Strategy for the Allied Health Professionals*. The Stationery Office, London.

DoH/DfEE (1999) *Working together to safeguard children: a guide for inter-agency working to safeguard and promote the welfare of children*. DoH, London.

Driscoll, J. (1994) Reflective practice for practice. *Senior Nurse*, **13** (7) 47–50.

Edwards, M. (1999) The future of practice nursing. In: *The Informed Practice Nurse*, (ed. M. Edwards). Whurr Publishers Ltd, London.

Elkan, R., Kendrick, D., Hewitt, M., Robinson, J., Tolley, K., Blair, M.,Williams, D. & Brumwell, K. (2000) *The effectiveness of domiciliary health visiting: a systematic review of international studies and a selective review of the British literature*. Health Technology Assessment, vol.4, no.13

ENB (1991) *Framework for continuing professional education for nurses, midwives and health visitors*. English National Board, London.

ENB (1995) *Creating Life Long Learners: guidelines for the implementation of the UKCC's Standards for Education and Practice following Registration*. English National Board, London.

ENB (1996) *Shaping the Future: practice-focused teaching and learning*. English National Board, London.

References

ENB (1997) *Standards for approval of higher education institutions and programmes.* (October 1997). English National Board, London.

ENB (1998) *Report of Practice Placements Review Visits – Learning Disability Nursing May 1997–April 1998.* English National Board, London.

ENB (2000) *Networking in Learning Disability Nursing: A Guide.* Chiltern Press, Luton.

ENB & DoH (2001) *Preparation of Mentors and Teachers: a new framework of guidance.* English National Board, London.

Entwistle, N. & Ramsden, P. (1983) *Understanding Learning.* Croom Helm, London.

Faugier, J. (1992) The supervisory relationship. In: *Clinical Supervision and Mentorship in Nursing,* (ed. T. Butterworth & J. Faugier). Chapman & Hall, London.

Feigenbaum, E. & McCorduck, P. (1984) *The Fifth Generation.* Signet, New York.

Flynn, P. & Knight, D. (1998) *Inequalities in health in the North West.* North West National Health Service Management Executive.

Ford, P. & Walsh, M. (1994) *New Rituals for Old: nursing through the looking glass.* Butterworth Heinemann, London.

Foucault, M. (1983) 'Afterword'. In: *Michel Foucault: Beyond Structuralism and Hermeneutics,* 2nd ed, (eds H.L. Dreyfus & P. Rabinow). University of Chicago Press, Chicago.

Fox, N.J. (1999) *Beyond Health: Postmodernism and Embodiment.* Free Association Books, London.

Franklin, B. (ed.) (1995) *The Handbook of Children's Rights: comparative policy and practice.* London, Routledge.

Gagne, R.M. (1970) *The Conditions of Learning.* Holt, Rinehart and Winston, New York.

Gerrish, K., McManus, M. & Ashworth, P. (1997) *The assessment of practice at diploma, degree and postgraduate levels in nursing and midwifery education: literature review and documentary analysis.* English National Board, London.

Ghaye, T., Gillespie, D. & Lillyman, S. (2000) *Empowerment Through Reflection: the narratives of healthcare professionals.* Quay Books, Wiltshire.

Gibbs, G. (1988) *Learning by doing: a guide to teaching and learning methods.* Further Education Unit, Oxford Polytechnic, Oxford.

Gillings, B. & Davies, C. (1998) Evaluating student performance. *Nursing Times Learning Curve,* **2**(8) 8.

Girot, E.A. (1995) Preparing the practitioner for advanced academic study: the development of critical thinking. *Journal of Advanced Nursing,* **21**, 387–94.

Goding, L.A. (1997a) Can degree level practice be assessed? *Nurse Education Today,* **17**, 158–61.

Goding, L.A. (1997b) Intuition in health visiting practice. *British Journal of Community Health Nursing,* **2** (4) 174–82.

Goding, L.A. & Cain, P. (1999) Knowledge in health visiting practice. *Nurse Education Today,* **19**, 299–305.

Griffiths, J. & Luker, K. (1997) A barrier to Clinical Effectiveness: The Etiquette of District Nursing. *Journal of Clinical Effectiveness in Nursing,* **1**, p.221–30.

Halgin, R.P. (1986) Pragmatic blending of clinical models in the supervisory relationship. *The Clinical Supervisor,* **3** (4) 23–47.

Handy, C. (1993) *Understanding Organisations,* 4th edn. Penguin, London.

Hannigan, B. (1999) Education for community psychiatric nurses: content, structure and trends in recruitment. *Journal of Psychiatric and Mental Health Nursing,* **6**, 137–145.

Harding, C. & Greig, M. (1994) Issues of accountability in the assessment of practice. *Nurse Education Today,* **14**, 118–23.

Hart, E. & Bond, M. (1995) *Action Research For Health and Social Care: a guide to practice.* Open University Press, Buckingham.

Hawkins, P. & Shohet, R. (1989) *Supervision in the Helping Professions.* Open University Press, Buckingham.

Henwood, M. & Hudson, B. (2000) *Partnerships and the NHS Plan: Co-operation or coercion? The Implications for Social Care.* Nuffield Institute for Health, Leeds University.

Heron, J. (1990) *Helping the Client: a creative practical guide.* Chapman & Hall, London.

Hinchliff, S. (ed.) (1992) *The Practitioner as Teacher.* Scutari Press, Harrow.

Holloway, E. (1995) *Clinical Supervision: a system approach.* Sage Publications, London.

Home Office (1998) *Supporting Families.* The Stationery Office, London.

Home Office (2000) *Domestic Violence: break the chain. Multi-disciplinary guidance for addressing domestic violence.* The Stationery Office, London.

Hudson, B., Hardy, B., Henwood, M. & Wistow, G. (1997) *Inter-Agency Collaboration: Final Report.* Nuffield Institute for Health: Community Care Division, Oxford.

Hudson, R. & Forester, S. (1995) Community practice teachers; the way forward. *Health Visitor,* **68** (4) 140.

Hughes, R. (1994) A critical evaluation of the use of andragogical models in tackling social inequality in nursing education. *Journal of Advanced Nursing,* **20**, 1011–17.

Humphries, J. & Tonge, J. (2000) Looking ahead: a forum for the future of school nursing. *Community Practitioner,* **73** (12) 881–3.

HVA (1994) *Protecting the Child: an HVA guide to practice and procedures.* Health Visitors Association, London.

Inskipp, F. & Proctor, B. (1993) *The Art, Craft and Tasks of Counselling Supervision. Part 1: making the most of supervision.* Cascade, Twickenham.

Inskipp, F. & Proctor, B. (1995) *The Art, Craft and Tasks of Counselling Supervision. Part 2: becoming a supervisor.* Cascade, Twickenham.

ILO (1985) *Convention 161. Annex B. Recommendation 171 concerning Occupational Health Services.* International Labour Organization, Geneva.

Jackson, C. (1994) PREP prompts cheers and fears. *Health Visitor,* **67** (4) 123.

Jardine, J. & Asherton, J. (1992) Development of community practice teaching in Swindon. *Health Visitor,* **65**, 88–9.

Jarvis, P. (1983) *Professional Education.* Croom Helm, London.

Jarvis, P. & Gibson, S. (1985) *The Teacher Practitioner in Nursing, Midwifery and Health Visiting.* Chapman & Hall, London.

Jarvis, P. & Gibson, S. (1997) *The Teacher Practitioner in Nursing, Midwifery and Health Visiting,* (2nd edn). Thornes, Cheltenham.

Jenkins-Clarke, S., Carr-Hill, R., Dixon, P. & Pringle, M. (1997) *Skill Mix in Primary Care.* Centre for Health Economics, University of York.

Jinks, A.M. & Morrison, P. (1997) The role of the external examiner in the assessment of clinical practice. *Nurse Education Today,* **17**, 408–12.

Johns, C. (1994) Guided Reflection. In: *Reflective Practice in Nursing: the growth of the professional practitioner,* (eds A. Palmer, S. Burns & C. Bulman). Blackwell Scientific, Oxford.

Johns, C. (1995) Framing learning through reflection within Carper's fundamental ways of knowing. *Journal of Advanced Nursing,* **22**, 226–34.

Jukes, M. (1994a) Development of the Community Nurse in Learning Disability: 1. *British Journal of Nursing,* **3** (15) 779–83.

References

Jukes, M. (1994b) Development of the Community Nurse in Learning Disability: 2. *British Journal of Nursing*, **3** (16) 848–52.

Kadushin, A. (1968) Games people play in supervision. *Social Work*, **13** (3).

Kadushin, A. (1992) *Supervision in Social Work*, 3rd edn. Columbia University Press, New York.

Kenworthy, N. & Nicklin, P. (1989) *Teaching and Assessing in Nursing Practice: an experiential approach*. Scutari Press, London.

Kirk, S. & Glendinning, C. (1998) Trends in community care and patient participation: implications for the roles of informal carers and community nurses in the United Kingdom. *Journal of Advanced Nursing*, **28** (2) 370–81.

Kloss, D. (1994) *Occupational Health Law*. Blackwell Science, Oxford.

Knowles, M. (1990) *The Adult Learner: a neglected species*, 4th edn. Gulf Publishing, Houston.

Krueger, R.A. (1994) *Focus Groups: A practical guide for applied research*, 2nd edn. Sage, London.

Le Grand, J. (1990) *Quasi-Markets and Social Policy*. Studies in Decentralisation and Quasi-Markets, No.1, School for Advanced Urban Studies, University of Bristol.

Linehan, M.M., Armstrong, H.E., Suarez, A., Allmon, A. & Heard, H.L. (1991) Cognitive behavioural treatment of chronically parasuicidal borderline patients. *Archives of General Psychiatry*, **38**, 1060–64.

Ling, M.S. & Luker, K. (2000) Protecting children: intuition and awareness in the work of health visitors. *Journal of Advanced Nursing*, **32** (3) 572–9.

Lipsky, M. (1980) *Street Level Bureaucracy: dilemmas of the individual in public service*. Russel Sage Publications, London.

Lowry, M. (1997) Using learning contracts in clinical practice. *Professional Nurse*, **12** (4) 280–83.

Lunt, N. & Atkin, K. (1999) The emergence and development of practice nursing – implications for future policy and practice. In: *Evaluating Community Nursing* (eds K. Atkin, N. Lunt & C. Thompson). Baillière Tindall, London.

Maggs, C. & Purr, B. (1989) *An Evaluation of the Education and Preparation of Fieldwork and Practical Work Teachers in England*. West London Institute of Higher Education.

Manchester Metropolitan University (2000) *Specialist Practice – 1: Practice Assessment Document; 2: Practice Learning Portfolio*. Department of Health Care Studies, the Manchester Metropolitan University.

Mander, G. (1997) Supervision of supervision: specialism or new profession? *Psychodynamic Counselling*, **25** (3), 291–301.

Marson, S. (1990) Creating a climate for learning. *Nursing Times*, **86** (17) 53–5.

Marton, F. & Saljo, R. (1984) Approaches to learning. In: A relational view of learning, (J. Cust (1996)). *Nurse Education Today*, **16**, 256–66.

McAllister, L., Lincoln, M., McLeod, S. & Maloney, D. (1997) *Facilitating Learning in Clinical Settings*. Thornes, Cheltenham.

MacDonald, A.L., Langford, I. & Boldero, N. (1997) The future of community nursing in the UK. *Journal of Advanced Nursing*, **26**, 257–65.

McHale, C. (1998) ENB Higher Award: evaluation of its impact on practice. *Nursing Standard*, **72** (12) 392–5.

MacLellan, M. (1996) Assessing practice: creative partnerships in action. *British Journal of Community Health Nursing*, **1** (8) 454–60.

McMahon, L. (2000) *Leading the Future: a report on a simulation based enquiry into the future of health visiting*. Community Practitioners and Health Visitors Association.

Maxwell, R. (1984) Quality assessment in health. *British Medical Journal*, **288**, 1470–72.

Melia, K. (1987) *Learning and Working: the occupational socialisation of nurses*. Tavistock, London.

Messick, S. (1976) Individuality in Learning. In: *Styles of Learning and Teaching*. (1981) (ed. N. Entwistle), p. 102. Wiley, Chichester.

Meizerow, J. (1981) A critical theory of adult learners. *Studies in Adult Learning*, **32**, 3–24.

Morriss, J. (1994) Community care or independent living. *Critical Social Policy*, **40**, 124–45.

Muir, J. & Sidey, A. (2000) *Textbook of Community Children's Nursing*. Baillière Tindall, London.

Neill, S.J. & Muir, J. (1997) Educating the new community children's nurse: challenges and opportunities? *Nurse Education Today*, **17**, 7–15.

Nursing Times Learning Curve (1999) Understanding how people learn. *Nursing Times Learning Curve*, **3** (5) 12–15.

Nyatanga, L. & Bamford, M. (1990) Mentorship scheme using the experiential taxonomy. *Senior Nurse*, **10** (5) 13–15.

Nyatanga, L., Walker, I.M. & Brooke, P. (1989) Facilitating the self care concept using the experiential taxonomy: Orem hires ET. *Senior Nurse*, **9** (2) 10–11.

Nyiri, J. (1988) Tradition and practical knowledge. In: *Practical Knowledge*, (eds J. Nyri & B. Smith). Croom Helm, London.

Oldman, C. (1999) An evaluation of health visitor education in England. *Community Practitioner*, **72** (12) 392–5.

Orlans, V. & Edwards, D. (1997) Focus and process in supervision. *British Journal of Guidance and Counselling*, **25** (3) 409–15.

Ottewill, R. & Wall, A. (1990) *The Growth and Development of the Community Health Services*. Business Education Publishers Limited, Sunderland.

Papp, P. (1983) *The Process of Change*. The Guildford Press, New York.

Parkes, K.R. (1984) Locus of control, cognitive appraisal and coping in stressful episodes. *Journal of Personality and Social Psychology*, **46**, 655–68.

Pearson, P. Graney, A. McRae, G. Reed, J. & Johnson, K. (2000) *Evaluation of the Developing Specialist Practitioner Role in the Context of Public Health. ENB Research Highlights*. English National Board, London.

Phillips, T., Schostak, J., Bedford, H. & Robinson, J. (1993) *Assessment of Competencies in Nursing and Midwifery Education and Training (the ACE Project)*. English National Board, London.

Poulton, B. (1997) *Practice Nursing: a changing role to meet changing needs*. Department of Health, London.

Power, S. (1999) *Nursing Supervision: a guide for clinical practice*. Sage, London.

Price, V. (1999) Psychosocial interventions: the organisational context. *Mental Health Nursing*, **19** (6) 23–7.

Proctor, B. (1991) On being a trainer. In: *Training and Supervision for Counselling in Action* (eds W. Dryden & B. Thorne). Sage, London.

Proctor, S., Campbell, S., Biott, C., Edward, S., Redpath, N. & Moran, M. (1999) *Preparation for the Developing Role of the Community Children's Nurse*. English National Board, London.

QAA (1997) *Subject Review Handbook*. Quality Assurance Agency, London.

Quinn, F.M. (1995) *The Principles and Practice of Nurse Education*, 3rd edn. Chapman and Hall, London.

Reed, J. & Procter, S. (1993) *Nurse Education: a reflective approach*. Edward Arnold, London.

Reynolds, S. (2000) The anatomy of evidence-based practice: principles and methods. In: *Evidence-Based Practice: a critical appraisal*, (eds L. Trinder & S. Reynolds). Blackwell Science, Oxford.

Rittel, H.W.J. & Webber, M. (1973) 'Dilemmas in a general theory of planning', Policy Sciences cited by M. Clarke & J. Stewart (2000) *Handling the Wicked Issues*. In: *Changing Practice in Health and Social Care*, (C. Davies, L. Finlay, A. Bullman). The Open University/Sage Press, London.

Robinson, G., Beaton, S. & White, P. (1993) Attitudes towards practice nurses: survey of a sample of GPs in England and Wales. *British Journal of General Practice*, **109**, 337–45.

Robotham, A. (2000) Health visiting: specialist and higher level practice. In: *Health Visiting: Specialist and Higher Level Practice*, (eds A. Robotham & D. Sheldrake). Churchill Livingstone, London.

Robotham, A. & Sheldrake, D. (eds) (2000) *Health Visiting: Specialist and Higher Level Practice*. Churchill Livingstone, London.

Rogers, C. (1969) *Freedom to Learn*. Merrill, Ohio.

Rowntree, D. (1987) *Assessing Students: how shall we know them?* Kogan Page, London.

Sackett, D.L., Richardson, W.S., Rosenburg, W. & Haynes, R.B. (1997) *Evidence-Based Medicine: How to Practice and Teach EBM*. Churchill Livingstone, New York.

Sadler, C. (1991) Schooled in Health. *Nursing Times*, **87** (23) 16–17.

Schön, D. (1987) *Educating the Reflective Practitioner*. Jossey-Bass, San Francisco.

Schön, D. (1990) *The Reflective Practitioner: how professionals think in action*. Basic Books, New York.

Schön, D. (1991) *The Reflective Practitioner*, 2nd edition. Arena Avonbury.

Shuldham, C. (1997) The leadership challenge in nursing. *Nursing Management*, **3** (10) 14–17.

Smith, A. & Russell, A. (1991) Using critical incidents in nurse education. *Nurse Education Today*, **11**, 264–91.

Smith, A. & Russell, A. (1993) Critical incident analysis. In *Nurse Education: a reflective approach* (eds J. Reed & S. Procter). Edward Arnold, London.

Somers-Smith, M.J. & Race, A.J. (1997) Assessment of clinical skills in midwifery: some ethical and practical problems. *Nurse Education Today*, **17**, 449–53.

Steinaker, N. & Bell, R. (1979) *The Experiential Taxonomy: a new approach to teaching and learning*. Academic Press, London.

Stoltenberg, C.D. & Delworth, U. (1987) *Supervising counsellors and therapists: a development approach*. Jossey-Bass, San Francisco.

Taylor, B. (1998) Locating a phenomenological perspective of reflective nursing and midwifery practice by contrasting interpretative and critical reflection. In *Transforming Nursing through Reflective Practice* (eds C. Johns & D. Freshwater). Blackwell Science, Oxford.

Tilley, S. (1997) *The Mental Health Nurse: views of practice and education*. Blackwell Science, Oxford.

Titchen, A. & Binnie, A. (1995) The art of clinical supervision. *Journal of Clinical Nursing*, **4**, 327–34.

Trinder, L. & Reynolds, S. (2000) *Evidence-based Practice: a Critical Appraisal*. Blackwell Science, Oxford.

Twinn, S. & Cowley, S. (1992) *The Principles of Health Visiting: an examination*. Health Visitors Association, London.

UKCC (1992a) *Scope of Professional Practice.* UKCC, London.

UKCC (1992b) *Code of Professional Conduct.* UKCC, London.

UKCC (1994) *The Future of Professional Practice: the Council's standards for education and practice following registration.* UKCC, London.

UKCC (1998) *Standards for Specialist Education and Practice.* UKCC, London.

UKCC (1999) *Practitioner-client relationships and the prevention of abuse.* UKCC, London.

UKCC (2000a) *Standards for the preparation of teachers of nursing, midwifery and health visiting.* UKCC, London.

UKCC (2000b) *The Nurses, Midwives and Health Visitors (Training) Amendment Rules Approval Order 2000.* website: www.hmso.gov.uk/si/si2000/20002554.htm

Ungerson, C. (1997) Social Politics and the Commodification of Care. *Social Politics,* **4** (3) 362–82.

UNN (1997) *Educational Audit Tool for Community Placement Areas.* University of Northumbria at Newcastle.

UNN (1999a) *University of Northumbria at Newcastle University Plan 1999–2000.* University of Northumbria at Newcastle.

UNN (1999b) *Roles and Responsibilities of External Examiners.* University of Northumbria at Newcastle.

Webb, B. (1997) Auditing a clinical supervision training programme. *Nursing Standard,* **11** (34) 34–9.

West, M. & Poulton, B. (1997a) Primary Health Care Teams: in a league of their own. In: *Promoting Teamwork in Primary Care,* (eds P. Pearson and J. Spencer). Edward Arnold, London.

West, M. & Poulton, B. (1997b), A failure of function: teamwork in primary health care. *Journal of Inter-Professional Care,* **11** (2) 205–12.

White, E. (1990) The historical development of the educational preparation of CPNs. In: *Community Psychiatric Nursing: a research perspective* (ed. C. Brooker). Chapman and Hall, London.

Wilding, P. (1992) The British welfare state: Thatcherism enduring legacy. In: *Policy and Politics,* **20** (3) 201–12.

Wiles, R. & Robison, J. (1994) Teamwork in Primary Care: the views and experiences of nurses, midwives and health visitors. *Journal of Advanced Nursing,* **20**, 324–30.

Wilkie, K. (2000) The nature of problem-based learning. In: *Problem-based Learning in Nursing – A new model for a new context* (eds S. Glen & K. Wilkie). MacMillan Press, London.

Wilkin, P. (1998a) Clinical supervision and community psychiatric nursing. In: *Clinical Supervision and Mentorship in Nursing,* 3rd edn, (eds T. Butterworth, J. Faugier & P. Burnard). Thornes, Cheltenham.

Wilkin, P. (1998b) *Clinical Supervision: the Rochdale support and development model.* Rochdale Healthcare NHS Trust, Rochdale.

Wilkin, P. (1999) Supportive supervision as a means of enabling self-awareness. *Nursing Times Learning Curve,* **3** (3) 10–11.

Wilkin, P., Bowers, L. & Monk, J. (1997) Clinical supervision: managing the resistance. *Nursing Times,* **93** (8) 48–9.

Williams, I.D.I. (1992) Supervision: a new word is desperately needed. *Counselling* **3** (2) 96.

Winter, A. & Teare, J. (1997) Construction and application of paediatric community nursing services. *Journal of Child Health Care,* **1** (1) 24–9.

Wong, J. & Wong, S. (1987) Towards effective clinical teaching in nursing. *Journal of Advanced Nursing,* **12**, 505–13.

References

Wood, N., Farrow, S. & Elliott, B. (1994) A review of primary health care organisation. *Journal of Clinical Nursing,* **3**, 243–50.

Wood, R. (2000) *From Data to Wisdom – can information and communication technologies finally deliver?* Inaugural lecture, University of Salford.

Yegdich, T. (1998) How not to do clinical supervision in nursing. *Journal of Advanced Nursing,* **28** (1) 193–202.

Yegdich, T. (1999) Lost in the crucible of supportive clinical supervision: supervision is not therapy. *Journal of Advanced Nursing,* **29** (5) 1265–75.

Index

adult learning, *see* learning approaches

andragogy, *see* learning approaches

assessment, patient/client, 35–7, 147, 178, 185

assessment, 68, 85–101, 130–31, *see also* specialist practitioner roles

  academic level, 95–6

  competency, 35, 87, 88, 97, 99, 128, 146, 148, 150, 162, 171

  concerns, 85, 87, 89, 92, 99, 137–8

  continuous, 88–90, 115, 164, 171

  critical discourse, 93, 115, 149, 164, 170

  diagnostic, 44–5, 90–92, 138, 144, 162, 163

  discussion, *see* critical discourse in assessment

  documentation, 137, 149

  equity, 85, 86, 97

  evidence, 87, 97, 98, 114, 115, 130, 149

  examinations, tests and essays, 90

  feedback, 67, 86, 87, 89, 98, 149

  formative (developmental), 87, 89, 98, 138, 184

  hidden agenda, 36–7

  individuality *see* interpersonal in assessment

  initial, *see* diagnostic in assessment

  interpersonal skills, 88, 148, 149

  learning contract, 94, 138, *see also* contracts in learning

  Manchester Metropolitan University assessment of practice, 96–8

  marking (grading), 96–8

  objectivity/subjectivity, 86, 95, 148, 149

  observation, 92–3, 115, 128, 149

  portfolio, 96–98, 98–100, 115

  reliability and validity, 95, 99

  self-assessment, 39, 93, 94–5, 98, 138

  significant others, 93, 130

  standards, 86–7

  summative (final), 87–8, 90, 98, 170

  timing, 37, 138

  tripartite arrangements, 138, 187, 149

  University of Northumbria at Newcastle assessment of practice, 98–100

audit, *see* audit(s) in quality

behavioural approach, *see* learning approaches

care and programme management, 4, 136

change, 12–13, 77, 78, 107, 112, 159, 160, 165, 195, *see also* clinical practice development, *see also* health service policy

clinical audit, 160, *see also* audit of practice in quality

clinical effectiveness, 50

clinical governance, *see* health service policy

clinical nursing practice, 4, 10, 77, 88–9, 91–2, 106, 112, 115, 156

clinical practice development, 4, 63, 77–83, 107, 117, 134, 160–61, 166–7, 176–7, 178, 193–4, *see also* health service policy

clinical practice leadership, 3, 4, 16, 18, 19, 95, 160

  development, 39–40, 41, 76, 117, 161, 164, 177

clinical supervision, 8, 37, 40, 54, 62–75, 94, 114, 120, 122, 123, 130, 148–9, 157, 181, 187

  assessment and supervision, 68–9

  boundaries, 66–7

  case work moments, 72

  definitions, 62–3

  educational, 63–4, 152

  functions, 63

power/empowerment, 66–8
prerequisites, 65–7
reflective model, 71–3, *see also*
    reflection
standards and audit, 65
supervision for the mentor, 73–4, *see*
    also support in mentorship
supervisory relationship, 63, 65, 69–71
transference and counter-transference,
    69–71, 75
cognitive approach, *see* learning
    approaches
collaborative practice, *see* partnerships
community care, 10, 13
Community Children's Nursing, 132–9
    mentor experiences, 133-6
    student assessment, 137–8
community health needs analysis, 15–16,
    18, 78, 79, 81, 113, 197
Community Learning Disability Nursing,
    10, 88–9, 125–131
    non-mandatory status, 126–7
    organisational context, 125–8
    student assessment, 130–31
    student experience, 128–30
Community Mental Health Nursing, 8, 94,
    118–24
    mentor perspectives, 122–3
    non-mandatory status, 119–21
    role, 118, 121–2
    student perspectives, 123–4
Community Practice Teacher, 7, 180, *see*
    also mentorship
competency, 35–8, *see also* competency
    in assessment
    enabling competence, 35–8
continuing professional development,
    134, 153, 192, 197–8, *also see*
    needs in mentorship
courses, *see* programmes in education
critical incident, 51, 78, 100, 137
    analysis, 53–9, 79
critical thinking, 10, 34, 93, 108, 115,
    123–4, 145, 148, 162, 164, 177
curriculum, *see* programmes in education

District Nursing, 7, 8, 56–9, 92–3, 108,
    135, 159–65, 173
    Audit Commission, 159, 160–61
    facilitating learning, 162–5
    role development, 159–62

SWOT analysis, 163

education,
    academic structure, 192–3
    accountability, 21
    commissioning, 21, 27–8, 112, 178
        funding, 8–9, 112, 119, 127, 194
        workforce development
            confederation, 21, 24, 27, 112, 127
    inter-professional, 192–3, 198
    links with practice, 27–8, 78, 84, 100,
        114, 131, 177, 193
    programmes, 26, 48, 173
        academic level, 5
        constraints, 84
        course organisation, 5, 173, 175–6,
            192–3
        curriculum, 44, 77–8, 86, 137, 140,
            191
        curriculum development, 23, 24, 27,
            191, 198–9
        ENB approval, 24, 26
        length of courses, 116, 140, 146, 170
        specialist practice, 4–5, 12, 18–20,
            38, 77–8, 142, 177–8, 191, 198–9,
            see also curriculum in education
        validation, 22–3
        viability, 126
    variation, 5, 19
educational theory *see* learning
    approaches
employment of mentors, 28, 65, 111, 112,
    125, 126, 131, 153–4
    organisational influences, 5–6, 111–14,
        116
    organisational structures and
        boundaries, 192–3, 111–12, 123,
        161
empowerment, *see* power
English National Board(s)
    annual monitoring review, *see* ENB
        review in quality
    Framework for Mentors and Teachers
        (2001), xvii, 7, 9, 193
    Higher Award, 76–84, 176–7
    standards, 4, 8, 23, 35, 86
evidence based practice, 16, 59, 105–7,
    165
    development, 105–6
    evidence based medicine, 105
    evidence based nursing, 105, 106

experiential taxonomy, *see* learning
approaches
external examiners, *see* quality

facilitation of learning, *see* mentorship,
see also District Nursing, *see also*
General Practice Nursing, *see also*
Health Visiting
field work teacher, 7, *see also* mentorship

general medical practice/practitioners,
13, 14, 56–9, 91, 111–12, 114, 141,
197
general practice fundholding, 13, 14
General Practice Nursing, 7, 35, 41–3,
90–92, 111–17, 173, 179
evaluating mentorship, 115–17
facilitating learning, 113–15
organisational context, 111–12

Health Act 1999, 14
health improvement programmes, *see*
health service policy
health service policy, 12–20, 27–8, 34, 68,
147, 150, 159–60, 188–9, 194
challenges, 192–5
clinical governance, 16, 18
development, 12–13, 16, 141, *see also*
clinical practice development
education, 12, 18, *see also* education
health improvement programmes, 14,
15, 16, 79, 113, 197
internal market, 13–16
National Service Frameworks, 16, 143
opportunities for learning, 77–83,
176–7, *see also* opportunities in
learning
political agenda, 13–14
Thatcherism, 13
the third way, 12
wicked issues, 189–91, 196–200
task force, 196
Health Visiting, 6, 7, 8, 10, 35–8, 81–3, 97,
135, 140–50, 173–9
facilitating learning, 143–6
policy context, 141–3
public health, 141–2,
student assessment, 148–9
vulnerable families, 146–8
higher award *see* ENB
higher education *see* education

Human Rights Act 1998, 139
humanism, *see* learning approaches

inter-agency work *see* collaborative
practice

knowledge acquisition, *see* learning

learning, 60, 63, 74–5, 122
constraints, 116, 182
contracts, 94, 113, 130, 136, 138, 162,
164, 184
diaries, 54, 60, 100, 164
experiential, 56, 58, 134, 155, 164
environment, 41, 44–6, 47–8, 63, 84,
85, 114, 130, 133, 134–6, 143–4,
152, 154, 162–3, 174, 175, 181,
191
evaluation, 80
evidence, 80, 82, 114
group work, *see* shared in learning
knowledge acquisition, 19, 51, 52
lifelong, 6, 8, 36, 116, 197–8
motivation, 38, 47, 67,
needs, 22, 34–5, 36, 64, 91, 94, 118,
120, 123–4, 142, 162, 163, 169,
180, 182
objectives/outcomes, 39–40, 79–80, 91,
96, 97, 129, 170–71
opportunities, 44–6, 89, 92, 135, 143–4,
163, 164, 171, *see also*
opportunities for learning in
health service policy
outcomes, 146, 170–71
portfolio, 97, 98–100, *see also* portfolio
in assessment
problem-based, 48, 59–60, 137
resources, 22, 29, 38, 47, 110, 128
shared, 53, 58–9, 119, 146, 175, 193,
199
skill acquisition, 39, 42, 43, 63, 91–2,
116, 121, 122, 136, 137, 142, 145–6
styles, 47–8
theory-practice integration, 5, 37, 48,
84, 86, 90, 120, 141, 145, 155–6,
164, 170
learning, approaches, 33–49
adult learning *see* andragogy
andragogy, 37, 38–9, 40, 42, 63
application, 49
behaviourist approach, 42, 43

cognitive approach, 42, 44
eclecticism, 42
experiential taxonomy, 155–7
humanist approach, 39, 40, 41
pedagogy, 38, 49, 63
postmodern theory, 136–7
relational theory, 47–8

managers/management, *see* employment
Mental Health Act 1983, 119
mentorship, xvii, *see also* specialist
    practitioner roles
    academic level, 5, 123, 126, 133, 174
    benefits, 134, 154–5
    clinical supervision, *see* clinical
        supervision
    community settings, xv, 6, 130
    constraints, 116, 153–4
    definition, 7, 168
    evaluation, 115–17
    flexibility, 46, 48, 116, 127–8, 133, 144,
        155
    historical perspectives, 7–8
    isolation, 117, 128
    knowledge and skills, 9, 108, 112, 127,
        171, 182, 183
    making a difference, 8, 10–11
    mentor–student relationship, 9, 39, 65,
        69-71, 91, 114, 116, 120, 123, 124,
        129, 136, 137, 144, 145, 169, 180,
        182, 184
    needs, 118, 122–3, 133, 134, 147
    non-mandatory status, 119, 120, 125,
        152–3
    practicalities, 113, 116, 123, 129, 164,
        183
    preparation, 6, 7, 125, 126–8, 129, 131,
        133, 167–8
    preparedness, 95, 126–7, 133-4, 174,
        178–9
    qualifications, *see* preparedness and
        preparation in mentorship
    risk taking, 183
    role conflict, 129–130
    role and responsibilities, 9, 10, 34–5,
        107, 118, 124, 136–7, 165, 167,
        171, 181, 184
    role modelling, 9–10, 108, 123, 164
    support, 45, 47, 73-4, 116, 120, 122,
        128, 129, 138, 168, *also see*
        support in clinical supervision

team, preparation and relationship, 47,
    113, 114, 121, 122, 144, 162, 181
tripartite arrangements, 36, 42, 86, 123,
    128, 129, 131, 135, 138, 154, 168,
    170, 184

NHS and Community Care Act 1990, 13
NHSE workforce development
    confederation, *see* commissioning
    in education

Occupational Health Nursing, 44–7, 70,
    97, 151–8
    employment issues, 153–5
    experiential taxonomy, 151
    placements, 44–5, 153–5
    role, 151–2

partnerships, 13, 86, 92, 112, 115, 145–6,
    189, 190
    inter-agency/inter-professional, 20, 77,
        108, 118, 145, 161, 192, 193,
    networking, 114, 138
    service users, 2, 28, 83, 107, 188–9,
        195
    team work, 56–9, 77, 93, 122, 136
pedagogy, *see* learning approaches
policies, *see* health service policy
power, 58, 162, 190, *see also* power,
    clinical supervision
practical work teacher, 7, *see also*
    mentorship
practice development, *see* clinical
    practice development, *see also*
    health service policy
practice educator, 7, 191, 198, 200
practice placement, *see* environment in
    learning
primary care groups/trusts, 12, 14–17,
    18–20, 19, 112, 113, 141, 161, 193,
    195
public health, 18, 19–20, 116, *see also*
    public health in Health Visiting
    community development, 15
    community participation, 141
Public Health Nursing, *see* Health Visiting

quality, 21–30
    audit (HEI), 22, 28–9
    audit of practice, 29, 65, 79, 127, 154,
        161

ENB review, *see* quality, professional and statutory bodies
mechanisms in HEI, 22, 23, 29-30
National Qualification Framework, 2
professional and statutory bodies, 21, 26–7, 127
quality assurance, 22–8
Quality Assurance Agency, 24–6
quality loops, 23, 29
subject benchmarks, 25–6

reflection, 48, 50-61, 74, 84, 90, 93, 137, 164, 170, 185–7, 190, *see also* critical incident analysis
historical perspective, 52
reflective frameworks, 53, 71–2
reflective practice, 71, 73, 120
structured reflection, 56
swampy lowlands, 121, 183
technical rationality, 52–3
relational theory, *see* learning approaches
research, 29, 52–3, 77, 79, 105, 106, 107–110, 133
research culture, 109–10
research in practice, 108, 145
research minded practice, 109

School Nursing, 10, 166–172
mentor preparation, 167–8
mentor-student relationship, 169
student assessment, 171
student support, 171–2
service users, 2, 28, 83, 107, 188–9, 195
skill acquisition, *see* skill acquisition in learning
skill mix, 6, 81, 82, 142, 193–4
specialist practice, 3-4, 9-10, 55–6, 71, 89, 106, 137, 193–4, *see also* specialist practitioner roles
specialist practitioner student, 19–20, 64, 180, *see also* specialist practitioner roles
academic level, 5
anxieties, 136–7, 172, 174–5, 185
autonomy, 38–9, 183
case loads, 127, 146, 163, 182–3
ENB standards, *see* ENB

expected outcomes, 4-5, 36–7, 38, 121, 146
funding, *see* commissioning in education
introduction to practice, 181–2
learning needs, *see* needs in learning
mandatory/non-mandatory status, 81, 111, 112, 118, 119, 120, 125, 126–7, 152, 166
motivation, *see* motivation in learning, personal social/domestic issues, 60, 66, 144–6, 172, 176
post-qualification employment, 6, 178
practicalities, 112, 173–4
preceptorship, 178
preparedness, 5, 6
prior experience, 91–2, 113, 114, 119, 120, 128, 134–5, 140, 144, 147–8, 155, 162, 169, 173
profiles, 113, 135, 162
responsibilities, 77, 82, 94
role transition, 113, 121, 127–8, 144–6, 162
satisfaction with education, 25, 29, 78
socialisation, 34
student–mentor relationship, *see* mentor–student relationship in mentorship
support, 40, 116, 149, 171–2, 179, 186, 187
specialist community practice, *see* specialist practice
standards
assessment, *see* standards, assessment
ENB, *see* standards, ENB
student, *see* specialist community practitioner student
SWOT analysis, *see* District Nursing

team work, *see* collaborative practice
theory–practice integration, *see* learning
transference/counter-transference *see* clinical supervision

UKCC policy, 3-6, 69, 77, 86, 142, 184

wicked issues, *see* health service policy
Winnicott, Donald, 63, 75